Integra
Person Care

Practitioner's Handbook

Tommaso Palumbo

Contents

Foreword

Following the success of Tommaso's first publication, I am even more enthusiastic with the foreword for this second work, as I have been witnessing my own clients improving their lives significantly by following the principles of Integrated Person Care.

Tommaso's strong affection for life and people - an enviable Italian characteristic that all of us can emulate - shines throughout his book. At once, we realize that life can be *more* than just manageable, but utterly pleasurable! With Integrated Person Care, we find the wisdom and the way to live a wonderful life. The source of this wisdom? Our own inner self!

We continuously search for the best guidance to help us 'win' in this complex and often disappointing world. Here, Italian passion for life embraces Eastern wisdom and Western knowledge, resulting in one of the most comprehensive and optimistic 'little' manuals on personal growth.

You are likely to find many answers to your questions in this book. Its principles and applications are bold and honest, making life much simpler than it often seems. Integrated Person Care can also be modified to fit the personal needs of almost anyone.

This guide is replete with theoretical and practical activities (*Pals* and *Bits*) to expand our vision of who we are and what we can do, and offers a gentle but persuasive plan for tuning up the personality and creating a lifestyle full of energy and hope.

Even if you have nearly given up on happiness, this book will convince you of your inborn potential to live a worthy life, one that is enriched with the things that count most, such as peace, understanding and love.

Tommaso acknowledges that existence is not easy, and asks us to face the challenges of living, squarely and intelligently. He has gathered some of the most significant theories of present and historic times, and offers a clear plan for the future that is second to none.

When reading this book, you are likely to feel as if you are in the company of a sage in the most comfortable of settings, soon discovering that all you need to know resides in your own being.

Tommaso's ideas encourage each of us to believe that we *can* make constructive changes and live a life that makes sense and matters, and that we *deserve* to do so.

In short, Integrated Person Care provides a distinctive map to reach the power within.

Read, enjoy, and follow the simple instructions of this book to find peace and joy in your life...*now*!

You will learn to believe in yourself again.

Dr Scott E. Borrelli
Chartered Clinical Psychologist.
Collegiate Professor, The University of Maryland, European Division.

Preface

I have been a Medical Practitioner now for almost twenty years and have always been interested in a holistic approach to my practice.

It was probably my interest in psychology that first attracted me towards medicine as a career, as a teenager. During my training I travelled to the United States to learn at first-hand about psychological and psychiatric interventions in California, where at the time many of their ideas remained based on Freud.

Throughout my training to become a General Practitioner, I embraced further training in counselling for varying stresses including bereavement and chronic illness.

I have always felt that medicine is both a science and an art, and that the complete person needs to be treated. I have no doubt whatsoever as a General Practitioner that addressing psychological issues can be as important as treating the physical manifestations.

I have known Tommaso Palumbo for several years now and worked with him with numerous clients. I think that a great deal of distress is generated by our modern high-pressure lifestyle at our places of work, in our social lives and in our personal relationships.

I have had extremely positive feedback from my patients who have seen Tommaso and have no doubt that his approach can be really beneficial for people suffering the rigors of modern life.

I feel, as someone once said to me, it is as important to relieve 'dis-ease' as it is to relieve disease and I believe that practising Integrated Person Care can significantly improve our physical and psychological health.

Dr David Parry

Acknowledgements

Dr Robert Lefever has kindly granted me permission to utilise a section of his book (*Eating Disorders*), which I have included in Appendix B. I would like to acknowledge that with gratitude.

I would also like to thank Dr Raffaele Morelli and Elisabetta Zerbini of Riza Institute, Rome, for a brief but very interesting and stimulating training experience.

A special 'thank you' to Margaret Russo, who has helped turn the original manuscript of this work into the current version.

I would like to thank Tina and Alberto Corsi of Borgo la Poggerina, la Romita (Tavarnelle Val di Pesa, Firenze) for the exquisite hospitality in their enchanting house.

Introduction
How to use this handbook

"There is the path of fear and the path of love. Which will we follow?"

Buddha *(1)*

Who is this handbook for?

This work has been developed with the purpose of being a useful guide for health care practitioners.

This guide could also be of interest to those who develop and manage health services. Fortunately there is, at present, an increased awareness of the value of preventative interventions and it seems that our policy makers have finally understood how investing now in preventative health programmes will save huge amounts of public resources in the near future.

However, I don't think that investing vast amounts of money in advertising campaigns urging us to eat more greens and fruit is the answer. Now, more than ever, we could benefit from programmes that are offered directly to critically important sections of our population. So, for example, offering person care training to university students or young parents will affect, at the same time, not just these groups, but their children and future generations.

The above interventions have more chances to be successful if they are:

> ➢ perceived as practically useful
> ➢ brief
> ➢ focussed
> ➢ easy to understand
> ➢ easy to apply

The Integrated Person Care (IPC) model has been created with the above characteristics in mind and, as a result, I believe that it may be employed as the core basis of a wide range of health care programmes.

This book could be a useful companion to every university student, regardless of their choice of studies. I look forward to the day when the first courses in IPC are introduced in our high schools and universities.

Finally, I am frequently asked if my approach would also be of any help to those suffering from mental illnesses (i.e. schizophrenia, bipolar disorders, etc.). I honestly don't know the answer to that question, as I have no experience of working with such persons. However, I think it would be appropriate to say that when these persons are going through a phase of relative normal mental functioning, they can benefit from some, or perhaps even all, of the activities recommended by my person care model.

Saying what I mean and meaning what I say.

The language we use to express ourselves is by no means a trivial matter. When some of us put on our 'professional hat', whether to write or speak, we may use technical words which could be difficult for outsiders to understand. Whole systems of professional power hang on to their privileges, and associated financial rewards, thanks to the jargon used, which normally sounds like a foreign language to most of us.

One way to ensure healthy sharing between humans is to use a language which is as clear and helpful as it can be.

I have also decided to throw political correctness in the bin, as too often it may prevent our communication from being open, direct and useful. I pull no punches and accept full responsibility for what I say here: having a choice between being, on the one hand, polite to fellow practitioners and respectful towards public institutions, and being, on the other, useful and helpful to sufferers of personal distress, I have no hesitation in opting for the latter.

The term 'practitioner' is used to refer to professionals working in the psychological field and to complementary health practitioners, while the term 'doctor' refers to medical practitioners. The term 'integrated practitioner' refers to professionals trained with us in Integrated Person Care (IPC).

When the term 'I' is used, I am expressing a personal opinion, whereas when the term 'we' is used, I am referring to consolidated research carried out on a particular issue. This is not an academic paper and, therefore, to keep the text flowing, I have preferred to avoid the continuous inclusion of detailed notes and references within the main text, wherever possible. Bibliographic sources, articles and research are duly acknowledged in the appropriate section of this handbook.

How to read this handbook.

This guide is divided into two main parts: the first introduces IPC, while the second presents its first level of application.

At the end of most sections you will find an 'Activities Box'. These boxes consist of two different sets of recommended activities, which I would encourage you to carry out before moving on to the next section if you want to make the most of this guided journey.

The first set of activities is called *PAL,* which stands for *Pondering A Little,* and offers food for thought exercises. The second set is called *BIT,* which stands for *Behaviour Improvement Training,* and provides a range of recommended practical actions.

So, you will be asked to spend some time with your *PAL* and to do your *BIT,* each step of the way. Do not rush through this guide as you would with an interesting novel which you cannot put down. Do not put pressure on yourself, even if you are really looking forward to the next step.

This is not a book to read: it is a book to interact with. Give yourself the time to go through each step thoroughly before you move on to the next.

If you are a qualified or a trainee practitioner, I would still recommend that you carry out all the exercises suggested in the activities boxes even if you feel that there are no particular personal issues you want to address. So, for example, when an Activities Box recommends to get in touch with a close friend or relative to find out whether they would be willing to be there for you and suggests to agree on mutually convenient times and ways to stay in touch, you can still get in touch with a friend or colleague and agree on a convenient time to discuss the recommended activity or, if you are really that busy, an exchange of emails would do.

Finally, please note that this brief work has three limited goals:

1. to illustrate how we can prevent and overcome some common forms of personal distress;

2. to introduce Integrated Person Care;

3. to present a person care programme whose well-defined step-by-step process would allow, and hopefully attract, further research on its effectiveness.

This book is not a treatise on psychological distress, nor does it offer a comprehensive account of the IPC approach.

At this stage of my professional development, I felt it appropriate to create this little tool to reach out to those sufferers or carers who would not otherwise benefit from the ideas and advice provided here, as well as to share my experience with those professionals who are striving every day to provide the best possible care within their own, often under-funded or under-staffed, work environments.

In other words, this work marks the starting point of what I hope will be a productive interaction with sufferers, carers and fellow practitioners. It is not meant to summarise a pre-existent debate, or offer conclusive statements about Integrated Person Care.

Getting started.

All you require to get started is the following:

- ✓ a pinch of motivation
- ✓ a one-week at a glance diary
- ✓ a few blank post-it notes (to be placed in the inside back cover of your diary)
- ✓ a notebook
- ✓ a pen or pencil

Make sure that you have all of the above with you before you start and … enjoy the journey!

PART ONE

~

INTRODUCING

INTEGRATED PERSON CARE

~

Chapter 1
What is Integrated Person Care?

"Blessings come from care, troubles from carelessness"

Buddha (1)

Cutting a long story short.

I have just hung up the phone. On the other end there was a lady who has been suffering from an eating disorder for many years. She told me that she was now desperate to do something about it, as her psychological distress and its impact on her professional and social life had become unbearable.

However, two concerns were still preventing this young lady from starting work on her issues. The first was to do with her lack of confidence in those professionals (i.e. counsellors, psychologists, psychiatrists) who were supposed to help her through the recovery process. She had seen a counsellor for some time and had not found her approach useful.

The second was about money. She had found out that practitioners specialising in eating disorders, especially those with more experience and better qualifications, were charging fees which were well out of her reach. She did visit her General Practitioner only to find out that there was a five months' waiting list to get an appointment with a psychiatrist on the National Health Service.

Luckily her mother was in a position to help financially. So, there she was, offering a brief account of her problems and enquiring about how I thought I could help her overcome them.

I have been seeing people in distress for over twelve years and have been receiving phone calls like the one briefly mentioned above almost on a daily basis for the past six years. The stories told and the resulting impact on people's lives may vary (i.e. depression, stress, anxiety, relationship difficulties), but either one, or both of the two main concerns expressed by the lady I have just spoken to – that is, a degree of diffidence or a lack of confidence in the psychological professions and a genuine concern about the cost of the service – have always been there.

Some do find, eventually, either the motivation or the financial means to seek and obtain help, but what had been troubling me for many years was the awareness that many more carry on experiencing considerable psychological pain, having their lives ruled by fears and obsessions without seeking help *simply* because of a lack of confidence in the 'helping professions' or because they don't have the financial means to obtain support.

It was six years ago, in January 2000, that I finally asked myself the following four basic questions:

1. Why do so many people have an issue with practitioners in the psychological field?

2. Why would so many spend their money on a new car or a new kitchen rather than invest it in their physical or psychological health?

3. Why is the 'know-how' of taking care of ourselves not freely, or very inexpensively, available to all those who would love to improve their physical and psychological well-being, but don't have the money to pay for it?

4. Is there anything I can do about it?

Activities Box 1.

Time for your *PAL* …
Get hold of a notebook and a pen. Sit comfortably somewhere and ask yourself the first three questions above. Write down your thoughts as you answer the questions.
Don't rush through your pal. Give yourself enough time to ask, think and write.

and for your *BIT*.
Go for a short walk around your office block. Walk slowly and see if you can notice something or someone that you had never noticed before. On your way back make a brief note of this experience.

Defining Integrated Person Care (IPC).

So, what happened when I asked myself the four questions indicated in the previous paragraph?

Well, you will find the answers to the first three questions as you progress through your reading of this handbook. When I asked myself the fourth question (*'Is there anything I can do about it?'*), to my surprise, a host of ideas started springing to mind: some old ones, whose value seemed worth investigating, and some new ones, whose practical application demanded to be tested in real life situations through my daily contact with people experiencing psychological distress.

That is exactly what I have been doing over the past six years and, as a result of the encouraging outcome of many interventions, I have created a new approach (IPC); I have founded a school which provides training in person care; and I am now writing this handbook, which will show you that there is so much we *can* do.

So, here we are ... sit back ... relax ... and, when you feel ready, let's have a look at what integrated person care is all about.

IPC is an independent territory whose natural boundaries are medicine, nutritional science, philosophy and psychology. IPC is an art, not a science: the art of healing the whole person.

Anybody can practise IPC as a way of life, regardless of their social background and religious beliefs. As you will shortly see, IPC does not clash with any moral norm, provided that you are a person of good will.

In IPC, we emphasise the role played by **sharing** and **prevention** in our well-being.

In common psychological and psychotherapeutic discourse the term *sharing* is associated with the private encounter between the psychologist-therapist and the patient-client within the confined space of a consulting room. It is a microcosm which, in the classic therapists' view, can adequately stage a comprehensive representation of the patients' macrocosm – that is, their real life, which comprises a given physical (home, car, office) and social (family, friends, colleagues) environment.

In its IPC connotation, *sharing* assumes the comprehensive meaning of utilising this actual meeting of two persons – the practitioner and the sufferer –

to help the latter widen their horizon and reconnect with their life forces in a different way by having the former fully engaged in the process: we call this 'sharing of inter-existential space', which means that the practitioner is wholeheartedly co-operating with the person.

As we will shortly see, most of the time there is absolutely nothing wrong with the person: it is their physical or social reality which would benefit from readjusting.

IPC shows the person how to go out there and create, or recreate, a web of meaningful relations – a precious resource of shared meaning – with their own environment.

Coming to the second term – *prevention* – we can clearly see how it has been utilised for some time now in medical discourse. Whether real preventative applications have followed or not, when it comes to our physical health, this is a matter we would be better not addressing here.

What we can observe, however, is that preventative measures are gloriously ignored by mainstream psychotherapy. We wait for a person to get deep into their distress before providing help. The service is provided when the client, often desperately, asks for it.

I don't share the above view of psychological help and I am convinced that there is a lot we can do to prevent our experience of personal distress, provided that we are taught how to take care of ourselves. This is one of the main goals of integrated person care.

IPC does not conform to the medical model of personal distress, whereby people are viewed as *patients* whose illnesses are treated by means of a given therapy.

In many cases people in distress do not require medication or long-term psychotherapy, as they may greatly benefit from a brief and focussed intervention involving bodywork, exploration of emotional issues and rational problems, education (training in emotional management and in helpful thinking), support and guidance.

IPC embraces the whole person. At first, IPC deals with our four components:

- physiological: our body and the physical sensations we get from it, such as hunger, headaches or pleasure;
- emotional: our feelings and the moods we allow ourselves, such as sadness, despair or happiness;
- rational: our thoughts and the state of mind we experience, such as worry, concern or understanding.
- behavioural: our actions as we practically express them.

Then, IPC works through our three dimensions:

- intrapersonal: our deeply rooted system of beliefs about us and the world;
- personal: our daily choices;
- interpersonal: the way we relate to others.

Finally, it addresses our three time perspectives:

- past: unresolved and resolved past issues;
- present: current issues;
- future: medium and long-term plans.

Over the past six years, my utilisation of the above approach has proved to be very effective in helping people who were experiencing different forms of distress such as eating disorders, anxiety, stress, depression and relationship difficulties.

Activities Box 2.

Time for your *PAL* ...
Note down your thoughts about IPC. What are, in your view, its strengths and its limitations?

and for your *BIT*.
Treat yourself to one healthy thing for each of the components mentioned above (i.e. physiological, emotional, rational and behavioural) and write them down in your notebook.

Chapter 2
Philosophical concepts

"Do not worry about tomorrow, for tomorrow will worry about itself."

Jesus (1)

"Live every act fully, as if it were your last."

Buddha (2)

Precious gifts from the distant past and from the near present.

The philosophical foundations of IPC owe much to the wonderful genius and inspiration of those who have dedicated their entire lives to the progress of human thought in their quest for wisdom. The least I can do is to briefly acknowledge some of them, and their contributions, here below, in chronological order.

I owe to **Taletes** (630 BC), father of the maxim 'know thyself' – which neither originates from Aristotle, nor comes from Socrates, though for some mysterious reason, it is generally attributed to the latter (3) – the gift of intellectual curiosity that I dearly treasure.

Journeying within ourselves can help understand better what goes on around us, while travelling around can help understand better what goes on inside us.

I am indebted to **Heraclitus** (circa 530 BC) for his concept of reality as a constant flow, which I have assimilated into my notion of change. The issue of change is an important one, as its understanding is one of the keys to good mental health.

When we see things as static, never-changing, we might be tempted into thinking that we can 'control' them. However, most of the time, our attempts at controlling reality fail miserably and when this happens, it hurts. We can avoid exposing ourselves to such unnecessary distress by appreciating how *panta rei,* 'everything flows', and, therefore, it would be more appropriate to focus our efforts on just being present to ourselves, being aware of reality, and doing our best to change it as we flow with it, rather than trying to control it.

Gautama Sakyamuni, '**Buddha**' (523 BC), has taught me the value and meaning of meditation. His view on the two goals of meditation – *samatha*, that is inner peace, and *vipasyana,* that is visual insight, intuition (4) – have been incorporated into my relaxation exercises.

His emphasis on peace and compassion as the most important factors for our well being (5), have been introduced directly into my approach to person care. I have found his reference to compassion particularly inspiring as the word itself evokes a combination of qualities (empathy, kindness, consideration, care) whose practical application into real life situations would result in healthy sensations, as well as helpful feelings, thoughts and behaviours.

Socrates (469 BC) has helped me give a new meaning to the usefulness of dialogue. I have learnt that when we engage in an open and direct dialogue, we are not simply talking to our interlocutor, we are also talking to ourselves and to the world, at the same time. This learning experience has contributed to the way I interact not only with persons in distress, but with everybody, in general.

From **Aristotle** (384 BC) I have borrowed the idea of three different and integrated 'souls' within each human being: his vegetative, sensitive and rational souls have become my physiological, emotional and rational components.

Another important concept I have learnt through him is that to 'know thyself' is not enough, if we want to achieve fulfilment and balance in our life (he would say 'to find what is Good').

The lesson I have learnt from Aristotle is that in order to 'find what is Good', to know thyself represents only the first step in the appropriate direction. The second step consists of the practical application of what we know about ourselves and to ensure that we follow our inclinations, which, in contemporary terms, would sound like 'be true to yourself in what you do with your life'.

I have assimilated the above into the 'dimensions' phase of the Integrated Person Care programme, where we explore and address our three dimensions: intrapersonal, personal and interpersonal.

Epicurus (341 BC) comes at the top of my very special list of great thinkers whose ideas have been mistranslated, misquoted and misrepresented because of bigotry, ignorance or political/professional interest (close second is Sigmund Freud, but we will talk about him later).

The first gift I have received from him is his invitation to relaxation and serenity thanks to a basic assessment of what really matters in life: his three categories of pleasure.

He placed first 'natural and necessary' pleasures (i.e. to nourish our body through eating and drinking, to protect ourselves against the elements), which is always appropriate to satisfy; second came 'natural but unnecessary' pleasures (i.e. to improve the quality of our food, to appreciate art and beauty, to make love), whose satisfaction is open to the question 'is this worth doing or not?'; third came 'non-natural and unnecessary' pleasures (i.e. to wear expensive clothes, to show off fine jewellery), which is never appropriate to satisfy because they are seen as a source of competition and envy, and, therefore appear to clash with healthy friendship among fellow human beings.

The second gift is the value of friendship. As he noted: "Friendship is the most precious amongst all the good things we receive from wisdom. Each morning Friendship goes around the world to awaken humankind, so that we can greet one another joyfully". (6)

The third gift is his view that "no one can come too early or too late to secure the health of his soul". (7) As Hadot observes, Epicurean healing "consists in bringing one's soul back from the worries of life to the simple joy of existing". (8)

As you can see, the medieval view of Epicurean thought as materialistic and hedonistic, which has been passed on to contemporary times, could not be farther away from the true meaning of Epicurus' message to humankind.

The truth is that while Socrates and Plato view the person as a citizen with their ethos and their duties towards their community, the Epicurean person was not a political entity to be fitted in a system of local or national organisations, but a simple and private human being whose main rule was to live in peace and harmony first with themselves and then with their physical and social environment. Such a message will always sit very uncomfortably next to dogmatic constructs like *nation, just war,* and *true religion.*

You will soon note how both the philosophical foundations and the psychological theories of IPC will draw from the above Epicurean concepts.

The teaching of the Stoics, from **Zeno** (332 BC) to **Seneca** (4 BC), and from **Epictetus** (50 AD) to **Marcus Aurelius** (121 AD), has given me an awareness of how focussing on the present moment can free us from the passions and troubles caused by the past and by the future, which do not depend on us.

As Seneca notes: "Two things must be cut short: the fear of the future and the memory of past discomfort; the one does not concern me yet, and the other does not concern me anymore." (9) The Stoics' concepts and practices of 'mental tension' and 'constant wakefulness' have been assimilated into the time perspectives' phase of my person care approach.

I have been brought up as a Christian and, naturally, the teaching of **Jesus** has greatly contributed to my personal and professional development. However, 'my' Jesus is the man who embraces people regardless of their race and faith with his warm and deeply human message of peace, love and understanding. This person would sit very uncomfortably – if he would sit, at all! – next to many clergymen that claim to speak on his behalf today.

Finally, from **Mounier** (1947), **Laszlo** (1978) and **Bellino** (1988), I have learnt about the logic of inter-existence, which I have fully embraced and which, as the following paragraph will show, constitutes one of the building blocks of the IPC philosophy.

"*To exist* – says Laszlo – *is more than to depend. To exist means to live and to act in the world as conscious human beings...aiming at our goals within a community based on interrelationship. The aim of inter-existence is growth and development; the means by which to attain it is an enlightened co-operation*". *(10)*

The above can be illustrated with a simple example offered by Bellino:
"*If I give you a coin and you give me a coin, how many coins have I got left? One. If I give you an idea and you give me an idea, how many ideas have I got left? Two*". *(11)*

Activities Box 3.

IPC philosophy.

The basic principles of the IPC philosophy are:

- we believe that our essence as humans – that is, our individual being – is unique and cannot be replicated;

- we are born neither good or bad and we direct ourselves towards one direction or the other depending on a variety of internal (i.e. genetic make up, faulty neuronal functioning) and external (i.e. upbringing, significant experiences, social contexts, traumatic events) stimuli;

- we believe in change and in its powerful impact on our development;

- we maintain that many generalisations (i.e. "people are like this, or people are like that") are inappropriate: *people* does not exist, millions of *persons* do exist, instead;

- we achieve peace – and, at times, happiness – when we nourish our essential needs, which may vary individually and are created as a result of internal (i.e. hunger or desires) or external (i.e. parental or social norms) factors;

- we nourish our essential needs when we get on the following virtual spiral: 'Peace through Development and Development through Peace';

- we reach Peace when we Develop as a result of keeping ourselves associated with our learning abilities and the life forces within and around us. We Develop as a result of being at Peace;

- we emphasise the role played by friendship in keeping us on the virtual spiral: friendship constitutes a powerful 'through' element between Peace and Development;

- we go beyond the logic of autonomy, which divides me from you, and the logic of interdependence, which makes you and me dependent upon one another, by opening ourselves to the logic of inter-existence. The logic of inter-existence is collaborative: it embraces me and you, us and them, and calls for an existence based on mutuality.

Activities Box 4.

Time for your *PAL* ...
Which of the above points do you agree or disagree with? Note down your thoughts about the IPC philosophy.

and for your *BIT*.
Which of the above points are you already practising in the way you talk and relate to others and which ones would you like to practise? Choose a suitable person and engage in a brief conversation about one of the above points. Afterwards, note down a brief account of the dialogue.

Choice and responsibility.

It has been observed how 'the view that human beings are defined by what they do is one of the key insights of Enlightenment thinking.' (12) It seems to me how, in recent times, we have lost the sense of the connection between what we do and the consequences of our actions. Persons are not held responsible for what they do and they blame everyone (i.e. parents, siblings, teachers) or everything else (i.e. poverty, bad weather) for their inconsiderate actions but themselves!

The basic fact that we are not accountable anymore for what we do and that we can even claim in our support behaviours that would be more appropriately counted in as additional proof of our full responsibility tells a lot about the state of our civic, political and judicial institutions. It would require a whole separate book to write on this topic, if the comprehensive social picture were to be taken into account. So, let's just focus on the psychological implications, on an individual level, of what is happening every day before our eyes.

Unfortunate persons, who, for their own protection, would better receive different consideration and attention, are gifted with a nice package of *'full choice and no responsibility'*. So we have cases when individuals suffering from severe mental illnesses are left free to go in and out of treatment centres at their pleasure, stab somebody to death, sue the state for compensation and win their case: the state knew about their illness and did not protect them from the emotional suffering of having killed someone.

The award of large sums of money as compensation to a murderer is outrageous when we consider that no financial support is provided for the victims of such crimes and that money does nothing for the mental problems of the perpetrator.

What is required here is proper care to prevent these situations from ever occurring again. Politically correct law makers have closed down psychiatric institutions because they were often found to treat the mentally ill inhumanely. So, rather than improving the quality of care and setting up a system of regular independent controls, politicians have simply opted for the cheaper alternative of releasing these persons into the community.

Our law makers have given a value to our life and it looks as if the life of ordinary persons like you and me is not worth much if they have preferred cutting on funds aimed at protecting our safety. Would things change if the next victim to be murdered by a known dangerously mentally ill person were a member of the royal family or one of the children of our beloved prime minister?

We are also graciously dispensing the same comfortable package of *'full choice and no responsibility'* to other individuals who would be better held fully accountable for their actions. Having been brought up in a poor family does not excuse or condone anti-social behaviour: the vast majority of poor or working class families are made up of honest and decent persons.

Excusing and condoning antisocial behaviour simply because it originates in a working class family is an insult to millions of persons who, like me, have been brought up in such an environment.

Likewise, running over and killing somebody while drink-driving makes the drivers even more responsible, because it was their choice to get drunk and not making use of other means of transportation. The same applies to persons driving while using their mobile phones. If you really deem it important to answer the phone or to make a call, you pull over and go ahead with it.

Only psychologically damaged societies, which keep in power inept or corrupted law makers, can allow driving while having a phone conversation. Do you remember life BC, Before Cell phones? How did we get along then? As far as I can recall, we were still able to run our own personal and professional life pretty well.

This state of affairs where full choice is not met with full responsibility is totally incompatible with the fostering of physical and psychological health. Irresponsible, but politically correct, law makers allow individuals to behave irresponsibly without having to worry about the consequences of their actions.

IPC would like to contribute to a new society where persons are first taught the meaning and relevance of basic personal and interpersonal behaviours and dynamics and, are then, either fully rewarded for their helpful input and sharing of experience, or fully held accountable for their anti-social choices.

Investing now in civic education programmes and, at the same time, in law-enforcement initiatives and effective alternative means of detention and rehabilitation, can save a vast amount of sorrow and money in the future. The sooner we realise this, the better for the physical and psychological health of our communities.

Activities Box 5.

Time for your *PAL* ...
What are your thoughts about the above point of 'choice and responsibility'?

and for your *BIT.*
Write down a brief statement of the principles which guide your behaviour, on a daily basis.

Chapter 3
Psychological theories

"If you can't find the truth right where you are,
where else do you think you will find it?"

Eihei Dogen (1)

The story so far.

Sigmund Freud viewed neurotic symptoms as 'the product of a conflict and a compromise between the primary unconscious impulses and the secondary conscious ones.' (2) As his daughter Anna clearly recalled: 'We felt that we were the first who had been given a key to the understanding of human behaviour and its aberrations as being determined not by overt factors but by the pressure of instinctual forces emanating from the unconscious mind.'(3)

From the early 1950s onwards many practitioners, especially in the US, started to grow increasingly dissatisfied with psychoanalysis and frustrated both with its passive nature and with the lack of tangible beneficial outcomes. First and foremost, among them, Carl Rogers and Albert Ellis.

Carl Rogers, arguably one of the fathers of humanistic psychology, published in 1951 his *'Client-Centered Therapy: Its Current Practice, Implications and Theory'*. In his view, the person is an integrating and self regulating whole, only when this balance is disturbed or incomplete do *dis-ease* (rather than *disease*) and dysfunction arise as symptoms, rather than causes.

Albert Ellis began developing a new approach – Rational Emotive Behavior Therapy, originally simply formulated as Rational Therapy – and established the Albert Ellis Institute in New York City in 1959. To clarify his views, Ellis uses a maxim of the Stoic philosopher, Epictetus (circa 50 AD). Epictetus noted how 'men are disturbed not by things, but by the views which they take of them'. (4) So, Ellis argued that it is not the event, but rather our interpretation of it, that causes our emotional reaction. He maintained that humans have a biological tendency towards irrational thinking (5), which in turns brings about painful emotions and self-defeating and unhealthy behaviour.

Another practitioner who took a critical stance towards psychoanalysis was Aaron Beck. He noted '...in psychoanalysis depression is caused by hostility turned against the self and anxiety is stimulated by the threatened break into consciousness of a taboo wish'. (6) He acknowledged how Freud's thesis that unconscious sexual wishes were 'converted' into hysterical symptoms ('conversion reaction') was the generally accepted one at the time. (7)

However, Beck did not surrender to the commonly accepted Freudian theses. He shared with Ellis the view that man's misconceptions of his life's events were the key to his emotional upsets and went on to propose that these incorrect conceptions originate in defective learning during the person's cognitive development. (8)

According to Beck, there are three different accounts for personal distress:

o the conditioning model (behavioural), where the stimulus (i.e. negative life event) leads directly to the emotional response;

o the psychoanalytic model, where the stimulus provokes an unconscious impulse, which in turn originates the emotional response;

o the cognitive model (Beck's own creation), where the stimulus meets a conscious meaning, which in turn triggers the emotional response. (9)

Finally, more recently, other mental health practitioners have been concerned not as much with what is going on inside our head (i.e. whether there is something wrong with us, and what is this all about), but, rather, with the powerful impact that external factors have on us. According to David Smail (10), many forms of psychological distress are the reasonable reactions of people to malign environmental circumstances. As Lerner and Sheldon also put it 'normal persons may experience abnormal events' and, as a result, it would be unreasonable to expect from these persons a normal reaction.' (11)

Naturally, we might debate what constitutes a 'malign circumstance' or an 'abnormal event'. However, what is interesting to note here is that the views presented above introduce an important shift from a traditional individualistic perspective, which maintains that when we are experiencing distress (i.e. feeling sad, lonely, stressed) it is us who require *fixing* and re-adjusting to the world, to a new social approach which suggests how it is the world which may require fixing and re-adjusting, instead.

As David Smail notes in his *How To Survive Without Psychotherapy:*
'Any adequate account of psychological distress, what causes it and what might alleviate it, must surely include the totality of our lives, and as part of that process take due note of the powerful, often inexorable, [social] forces that shape us in the world beyond the consulting room. Psychological distress, I am suggesting, is not a problem of the person or of the self, but is a problem presented for the person by the world.' (12)

Activities Box 6.

Time for your *PAL* ...
Which one of the three accounts provided by Beck sounds right to you? Note down your reflections.

and for your *BIT.*
Choose a suitable person and discuss the last topic addressed in this paragraph (i.e. 'do we require fixing or is the world that requires re-adjusting?'). Afterwards make brief notes of your conversation.

The human brain.

This paragraph is not about dispensing anatomical notions, which you are required to memorise and remember. I have just gathered here below a few useful references about our brain functioning because this will help you understand both the IPC explanation of personal distress and the guiding principles of its practical application.

We might not know enough about the key individual differences between our brains, in terms of their functioning, like why some people are better at a specific activity than others (13), but we have a pretty good idea of what our brain looks like and a growing body of knowledge is rapidly accumulating on how some parts of it work, thanks to the progress made in neuroscience.

Very simply put, our brain is made up of five parts. The bigger one consists of the well-known left and right hemispheres (telencephalon), while the other four are often referred to collectively as the brain stem – the stem on which the cerebral hemispheres sit. (14)

The cerebral hemispheres are covered by a layer of tissue called the cerebral cortex. About 90% of our cerebral cortex is neo-cortex, that is, new cortex of relatively recent evolution. (15) Beneath the neo-cortex there are several other sub-cortical groups or components (i.e. limbic system and basal ganglia) and among them the amygdalas – two almond-shaped nuclei. (16) The amygdalas are generally stated in the singular, however, please note that there is one in each hemisphere.

What I would like you to know is that the neo-cortex is our thinking brain (our true rational level), while the sub-cortex is our emotional brain. Most importantly, I would like you to appreciate that the latter was there long before the former developed. The cortex is the 'intellectual' part of the brain that controls such functions as problem-solving, planning, speaking. It is the cortex that is at work during psychotherapy. (17) However, as David Servan-Schreiber observes "it is the emotional brain, or limbic system, that produces the fear and rage that trouble those who are psychologically distressed and where memories of trauma and neglect are stored." (18)

We now know that our emotional memories are stored in the amygdalas. (19) The amygdalas are centrally involved in interpreting the emotional significance of experience.

As van der Kolk observes: "...the amygdala serves as the 'smoke detector' that interprets whether incoming sensory information is a threat. It forms emotional memories in response to particular sensations, sounds, images etc. that have become associated with threat to life and limb. These emotional interpretations are thought to be indelible, i.e. extraordinarily difficult to extinguish: once the amygdala is set to remember particular sounds, smells, bodily sensations, etc. as dangerous, the body is likely to respond to any of these stimuli as a trigger for the return of the trauma. The challenge of any effective psychotherapy, therefore, is to de-condition the amygdala from interpreting innocuous reminders as a return of the trauma." (20)

So, simply put, we do not benefit from over-active amygdalas, which are likely to get stuck with emotional association with past events and memories, rather than simply processing them.

Recent research has also shown an association between fast recovery in response to negative and stressful events and effective modulation of activation in the amygdalas. (21)

So, it looks like we don't benefit from under-active amygdalas, either. The challenge, therefore, is to make sure that the 'smoke detectors' in the amygdalas go off only for the time necessary for us to be aware of what we are experiencing – so that we can look after it – and then we want to re-set them to normal functioning.

I would like you to note that neuroscientists agree on the basic fact that "the harmonious integration of mental functioning starts at the level of the brain stem – a part of the brain that is essentially hidden from conscious experience, and cannot really be modified by reason." (22)

So, it looks like rational interventions alone are not able to fully reset our emotional smoke detectors when they go off. I hope that the above recent research findings provide some food for thought to those who believe that cognitive therapy alone is *the* answer to the problems which afflict humankind.

Finally, let's take a look at what the latest research can tell us about depression. The traditional view was that depression was caused by low levels of serotonin, the brain chemical which regulates our mood. In the late 1990s, psychiatrist Yvette Sheline carried out research at Washington University in St Louis which showed how the hippocampus (a region of our emotional brain) was up to 15 per cent smaller in women with depression and the longer each woman had been depressed, the smaller her hippocampus. (23) Depression is therefore more than a simple matter of depleted brain chemicals.

It had long been thought that new neurons are born only during brain development and that if neurons die during adulthood they cannot be replaced. But, in the late 1990s and within months of each other, researchers from two different teams – Fred Gage of the Salk Institute in San Diego and Elizabeth Gould of Princeton University – showed that the adult hippocampus can, in fact, make new brain cells. The brain damage seen in depression might not just be a result of cells dying, but also a lack of cells being born – a process called neurogenesis. (24)

How do we help the birth of our brain cells? A substance called BDNF (brain-derived neurotrophic factor) was originally identified as a 'growth factor' involved in the development of the nervous system, but it is now known to be important for sustaining and protecting neurons in the adult brain.

Ronald Duman and his colleagues at the University of Texas Southwestern Medical Center in Dallas, propose a 'neurotrophic theory' of depression, in which the antidepressant effects of drugs like Prozac could be attributed to the way they keep cells alive in the hippocampus. (25)

So, how do we help brain cells in the hippocampus re-grow? You may like to know that drugs aren't the only way to raise BDNF levels. Exercise, omega-3 oils and acupuncture can do it as well. (26) We will expand on this in the 'sensations' chapter of this handbook.

Activities Box 7.

Time for your *PAL* ...
Think about something you really like (i.e. a particular food, a piece of art). Note down what you like about it.

and for your *BIT*.
The next time you are stepping out of your front door, note down the first thing that you like. Do the same when you get back home.

The IPC explanation.

What is it that I do not find convincing in the psychological theories briefly introduced in the opening paragraph of this chapter, especially in the light of what we now know about our brain functioning?

I have the highest admiration for what Freud has managed to achieve in his lifetime and I truly regard him as a pioneer whose work and ideas have greatly contributed to the development of many disciplines. However, this does not change the fact that his theories are one hundred years old.

Moreover, psychoanalytic theories are like religious dogmas:

- there is no way to test them;
- scientific research is gradually and surely exposing their shortcomings;
- they can easily lead to abuses in the name of beliefs held as Truths by their most orthodox practitioners.

This is especially the case in the US, where analysts believed that Parkinson's disease, for instance, was supposed to stem from anger the sufferer could not cope with. George Gershwin's analyst declared Gershwin fell off his piano stool because he was hysterical. Gershwin had a brain tumour! (27)

Albert Ellis' practical approach to personal distress – Rational Emotive Behaviour Therapy (REBT) – is surely one of the most helpful and user-friendly created so far. However, when he says that we suffer from psychological distress because we have a biological tendency towards making our life a complicated mess, he does not add much to our understanding of what's happening to us when we experience psychological problems, and, as a result, sufferers may end up applying REBT's techniques mechanically to their situations. For how long will these quick and ready-to-apply fixes patch up the person's long-term emotional pain?

Aaron Beck, the father of Cognitive Therapy, notes: 'A significant difference between psychological disorders and normal emotional responses is that the ideational content of the disorders contains a consistent distortion of a realistic situation. Whereas the normal emotional response is based on a reasonable appraisal of the reality situation, the responses in psychological disturbances are determined to a far greater degree by internal (that is, psychological) factors that confound the appraisal of reality.' (28)

Now, as we have just seen in the previous section, when we have introduced the amygdalas and we have briefly mentioned some basic aspects of their functioning, the latest research shows how emotional distress is not caused just by rational 'distortions' or by a less 'reasonable appraisal of a reality situation'. The amygdalas (that is, our 'emotional smoke detectors') simply go off when incoming sensory information triggers specific emotional responses, which they have in store. Rational processes are simply not part of this movie, not even as extras!

So, for example, imagine that you have been attacked and robbed four years ago by somebody wearing a strong aftershave and, as a result, you did experience feelings of anxiety, fear, anger and helplessness. If you haven't reset your amygdalas, you may experience sensations of anxiety, fear, anger or helplessness just because somebody sitting next to you in the train today was wearing a strong aftershave! There is nothing rationally distorted about this!

It would be appropriate, instead, to acknowledge that, although we function as a whole unitary system, different parts of our system speak different languages (i.e. a physiological, an emotional and a rational language), which we are perfectly able to interpret and understand when we are in 'normal functioning' mode and totally incapable of making sense of when our 'smoke detectors' go off and cause us emotional distress.

As Servan-Schreiber observes: *"Neuroscience research has shown clearly that the basic disorders involving depression, stress and anxiety are all related to the functioning of our emotional brain, which we mostly do not understand and look after badly. The same research explains why concentrating on the body can be so effective. Besides producing emotions, the limbic system is also intimately linked with our major metabolic systems – the heart, the guts, the hormones and the immune system. There is constant two-way traffic, with messages coming up about what is going on in the body and messages going out to ensure a smooth working of the whole...This new picture explains why working with the body can be more effective than psychotherapeutic talking cures – the links between the emotional brain and the body are denser and faster than those between the emotional brain and the cortex."* (29)

We also know that 'the pain wiring of the nervous system is like a warning device that protects the body from tissue injury or disease. Acute pain is like a properly working alarm system: the pain matches the damage and it disappears when the problem does. Chronic pain is like a broken alarm: a wire is cut or hurt and the entire system goes haywire.' In such cases 'the repair doesn't occur because the [alarm] system itself is damaged.' (30)

The IPC explanation of emotional distress is based upon the new knowledge we have acquired through the research carried out on our neural functioning briefly indicated above, that is, that our emotional processing system (the amygdalas) when stimulated by certain sensory information may go off, just like two smoke detectors, to alert us that there is something or someone worth taking care of.

Is it appropriate to draw such a parallel between physiological and emotional functioning? I believe it is. As Thernstrom observes 'Pain and depression both share the same neural circuitry. The neurotransmitters and hormones modulating a healthy brain – such as serotonin, endorphins [and brain-derived neurotrophic factor] – are the same ones that control depression. Chronic pain uses up serotonin in the brain like a car running out of petrol. If the pain persists long enough, the petrol runs out.' (31)

So, in the vast majority of cases, there is nothing wrong with us! To the contrary, our perfectly functioning emotional detectors are simply drawing our attention to an internal or an external stimulus and to the basic fact that we may not have enough resources to deal with it, at that moment in time.

Therefore, all we want to do is to take care of the warning, reset the system and provide the required resources. Naturally, if we don't do that at the appropriate time and place and if we keep on ignoring our smoke detectors going off, we get to a point when the alarm system itself gets damaged and, eventually, we end up sitting in front of physicians or therapists, who believe that we are damaged (the whole person, not just our alarm system!) and will, in turn, listen to the full account of us presenting our symptoms, negative thoughts and rational *distortions*, and start *treating* them by means of medication, psychological therapy or a combination of both.

But are physicians and therapists assessing and dealing with the whole persons, or are they focusing on one or more of the many SOS signals that these persons are sending out, due to their problems? Do we believe that our issues can be properly diagnosed when we are in such emotional states?

If we were seated comfortably in a boat and a woman was drowning in the ice cold water three feet away from us, do we really think that that would be an appropriate time to have a productive conversation about this lady's upbringing, or about her relationship with her father or mother, or, perhaps to ask her about some of her latest dreams or some of her reoccurring negative thoughts?

The woman is drowning. There can be no *if* or *but* here, no grey area to discuss: do we throw a life buoy at her and help her to climb on board or do we throw at her a couple of inventories and a pen?

I know what I would do, and that is exactly what the Integrated Person Care approach is all about: helping people out of their emotional distress, first, before even contemplating more in-depth (analytical or cognitive) work, which could prove utterly unnecessary, if not even damaging to the person, at an early stage of their recovery.

I believe that when we ignore the warning coming from our emotional detectors for a period of time, we enter a phase of *emergency functioning* where we are not our real selves anymore and we find it difficult to make sense of what is going on in our life, let alone to see the light at the end of the tunnel.

When we get into emergency functioning, our emotional selves get into survival mode: they shut down, create a social vacuum around themselves and wait for the remaining healthy parts of our system to start the resetting process.

I also believe that it is not just our emotional detectors' system that may enter a phase of emergency functioning. I think that the same applies to our body and to our rational mind when we develop an addiction to unhealthy habits or we are faced by worries and we don't deal with them at the appropriate time and place.

We already know that we have physiological sensors all over our body, like our satiety sensors that check if we have enough fuel to carry on. I am confident that neuroscience and medicine will discover the rational equivalent to what the amygdalas are for our emotional self. At this point, I would simply call them *rational sensors*.

Sometimes the reset is automatic, time is a healer, as they say, and not much is required on our part. However, in other circumstances we are required to do it by ourselves, manually, and that's when the trouble starts, because most of the time we think we know what to do and how to do it, when too often we don't have a clue, or we don't come across sensible advice, ending up making things even worse.

I believe that there are four components to each of us (physiological, emotional, rational and behavioural) and that it does not really matter which one of them got affected first by an unhealthy internal or external sensory stimulus, because in a matter of days, if not hours, the remaining three get affected as well.

That's why people with very different issues may display similar symptoms or why, to the contrary, sufferers from similar problems may present themselves with various warning signs.

If we decide to go down the 'symptom route', so dear to pharmaceutical companies and some academic establishments, then we may identify a different psychological illness for each different behaviour or symptom displayed. Of course, a new disease will require either increased prescribing of a given drug or a new medication altogether, all nicely sprinkled with some more research funding available for some privileged sections of the academic community: enough to keep a fair number of important people happy with their job and a few multinational drug companies satisfied with their business.

Not surprisingly, then, this is what is happening, before our very eyes, almost on a daily basis: professionals look and don't see, listen and don't hear, or, perhaps, it would be more appropriate to say that they selectively see what they want to see and hear what they want to hear, given that we keep on hearing of the continuous 'discovery' of new variants of psychological illnesses all the time.

As Dorothy Rowe acutely notes "The DSM lists some 39 different kinds of depression, including 'depression in complete remission'. You might think you are happy but your psychiatrist knows that the illness is still lurking there!" (32)

When people are going through a phase of emotional or rational emergency functioning they don't really know what is going on in their life, because for survival reasons they are temporarily disconnected from the remaining healthy parts of their system, whose task is to keep them alive at all cost.

Therefore, we can appreciate how creating elaborate diagnoses just on the basis of some symptoms or behaviours displayed, rather than shifting our focus on the whole person, could be either misleading, or inappropriate, or both.

I believe in the power of change and in personal responsibility. People can choose healthy, useful and helpful options or unhealthy, self-defeating and unhelpful alternatives. Most of the times, the choice is ours.

I don't believe in personality traits. I am much more interested in what changes over time *within* persons than in alleged individual differences *between* them.

Furthermore, who says that there is something wrong *within* the individual person? In many cases, what does set off the detectors has nothing to do with the person, but it is associated with how that person is relating to his/her physical or social environment.

It is either a case of addressing and improving interpersonal skills, or a case of making the person aware of how unhealthy some environments are and help them realise what they can do to change their current reality – rather than 'treating' alleged internal, biological, developmental or cognitive deficiencies.

My concerns about the diagnostic categories adopted in mental health and about the tools practitioners use to fit sufferers into one of them are shared by eminent practitioners and academics.

In a paper published by the Lancet, Prof. Fairburn and Prof. Harrison from Oxford University Department of Psychiatry write: "The existing scheme for classifying eating disorders is unsatisfactory and anomalous, in that about half the cases seen in clinical practice are relegated to an atypical or not otherwise specified group. This system is a historical accident that needs to be rectified, since far more unites the three categories of eating disorders than separates them. A classificatory scheme that reflects clinical reality would greatly facilitate research and clinical practice." (33)

By the way, do you know where the diagnostic categories used in psychological practice come from? They come from the American Psychiatric Association, that is, an organisation entirely made up of real and, hence, fallible, men and women: last time I checked there were no semi-deities among their members!

What I propose is to take care of resetting, in each case, all four components. Different approaches work differently for different people who are experiencing different phases of emergency functioning due to different internal or external stimuli. How do we know, then, which model could be more beneficial to some sufferers and less to others?

Only by addressing the whole person can we be reassured that we are guiding them on the path of a full recovery. That is what I have done, in my professional practice, over the past six years and the encouraging outcomes of my approach to some common forms of personal distress, such as stress, depression, anxiety and eating disorders, have motivated me to share here my working model with carers and fellow practitioners.

Finally, there is just one last point I would like to make. Freud has built a truly sophisticated and impressive theoretical construction to account for the way our mind functions and our neuroses originate, as a result of the dynamic interaction of 'I', 'Super-I' and 'It'. He has left rivers of regularly mistranslated and misinterpreted words on the topic. What about me?

Well, naturally I am not even remotely comparing myself to the great Austrian master – my ideas are likely to attract enough criticism as they are.

However, I would like to close this section by briefly mentioning what I believe goes on in our mind and I will keep it so short and simple that, hopefully, it will be very difficult to mistranslate or misinterpret my thoughts.

I believe that there are three co-existing components within our 'unitary' system (that is, one mindbodyspirit entity): the biological, the emotional and the rational. Together, they generate the fourth component: the behavioural one, which can, in turn, affect its 'parents'.

The biological self is the result of millions of years of evolution of our species on this planet. It has sensors all over our body to be able to detect any kind of discomfort (i.e. hunger, thirst, cold, etc.). It knows exactly what to do and how to take care of itself.

However, it can be affected by external sources (i.e. polluted environment, food poisoning, viral infection) or by internal ones (i.e. unhealthy, and, often, plainly stupid behaviours, unhealthy demands from the cognitive self like excessive work load). This is the element that we reset when we address our physiological component.

The emotional self is the instinctual, direct, raw and creative part of our system, whose experiences are stored in the amygdalas. It asks for immediate satisfaction and may either lead us to dark, sad and lonely places, or to sunny, happy and welcoming lands.

It can be affected by external sources (i.e. bereavement, loss or other traumatic events, stressful environment) or by internal ones (i.e. poor physiological care, like not eating or sleeping properly, lack of exercise, inner emotional conflicts). This is the element that we reset when we address our emotional component.

The cognitive self is the logical, indirect, more sophisticated and practical part of our system, whose information is stored in the neo-cortex. This is the element that asks for supremacy over the entire system.

It is the last we have developed, in evolutionary terms, and just like all newly-appointed masters, it thinks it is the smartest and knows it all. Not surprisingly, then, it may get really upset and frustrated when it realises, sooner or later, that it is not able to get very far on its own without the proper support of the other two components of the whole system. This is the element that we reset when we address our rational component.

Activities Box 8.

Time for your *PAL* ...
When you are experiencing psychological distress do you mostly feel it with your body (i.e. developing headaches or stomach aches), do you mostly feel negative emotions or do you mostly think negative thoughts?
Has it always been like that, or have you noticed a change over time either in the way you experience your distress or in the level most affected? Note down your reflections.

and for your *BIT.*
The next time you are stepping out of your front door, note down the first thing that you don't like. Do the same when you get back home. Then, observe your response.

Psychotherapy or Person care?

If Sigmund Freud were alive today I very much doubt that he would be happy about what happened to his creation – psychoanalysis – over the past sixty years. He wanted to create a new kind of practitioner, a 'Seelsorger' ('healer of souls'), a professional who was not a physician, nor a priest: in reality, the practice of psychoanalysis has been confined for many years, and until recently in the US, only to medical practitioners and psychiatrists. (34)

He, also, completely underestimated the value of having his works correctly translated into the English language, and understandably so. After all, when he was alive the official languages of culture were still French and German.

He could not foresee that, as a result of World War II, some of the best minds would emigrate from Europe to the US, and that the new American Empire was to establish the supremacy of its language.

The US had the means to invest in research and to carry out psychological studies that contributed to establish English as the official language of psychology too!

When somebody from his cultural and linguistic background would try and draw the old master's attention to the shortcomings of the translations of his works, he would benevolently say "I'd rather have a good friend than a good translator". (35)

I don't speak German and I owe the above insights to a little book by Bruno Bettelheim, 'Freud and Man's Soul', which I strongly recommend to anybody contemplating a career as a psychological practitioner. What I now know is that when we read passages from Freud's work such as "psychoanalysis is a procedure for the medical treatment of neurotic patients" (36), I am fully aware that Freud himself would have found it as cold and unconnected from human nature as I, and probably most of you, did.

As Bettelheim notes: '...of all the mistranslations of Freud's phraseology, none has hampered our understanding of his humanistic views more than the elimination of his references to the soul (die Seele). The word that the translators substitute for 'of the soul' – 'mental' – has an exact German equivalent; namely, geistig, which means 'of the mind', or 'of the intellect'. If Freud had meant geistig, he would have written geistig. It is true that in common American usage the word 'soul' has been more or less restricted to the sphere of religion. This was not the case in Freud's Vienna, and it is not the case in German-speaking countries today. In German the word Seele has retained its full meaning as man's essence, as that which is most spiritual and worthy in man.' (37)

As a result of the systematic mistranslation of Freud's work into English, a revised version of his theories and of his working model emerged, which was overloaded with cold and aseptic medical terms and references. The translator introduced words that had no connection whatsoever with human nature, that totally misrepresented Freud's original thoughts, which were warmer and permeated with profound humanity. It was such a mistranslated version that many eminent psychoanalytic practitioners used as the basis for their studies and training.

Other mistranslations include: 'mutterleib', the mother's womb, became the 'uterus'; 'zerlegung', taking apart in a cognitive way, became 'anatomy'; 'Ich', I, became 'Ego'; 'Uber-Ich', over-I, became 'Super-Ego'; 'grausam', cruelly, became 'shockingly'; 'versprechen', lapses, became 'slips of the tongue'; 'fehlleistung', faulty achievements, became 'parapraxis'; 'besetzen/besetzung', to occupy, occupation as in invested with psychic energy, became 'cathexis'; 'einfall', sudden idea, became 'free association'; 'trieb', drive, impulse, became 'instinct'; 'schicksale', fates, destinies, became 'vicissitudes'.

Given these premises, we are not surprised to find, even in contemporary psychodynamic practitioners, remnants of the same degree of detachment from human nature and scepticism in the human capacity for change that were displayed by psychoanalysts sixty years ago.

This is what Michael Jacobs, a leading figure in the psychodynamic approach, says as recently as 2002:

*"Working once a week with a person, rather than several times a week, puts some limits on the type of client who can be seen, although experienced psychodynamic counsellors often see clients who are as **damaged** as any seen by the majority of psychotherapists"... "Psychodynamic counselling involves condensing the psychoanalytic method; but this can be very taxing, because her or his psychodynamic training cannot help but make the counsellor aware just how complex the human personality is, and just how **slow the process of change is.**" (38)*

So, what do you think? Do you share the above view that quantity equals quality, that in order to carry out decent person care work you are required to see your practitioner several times during the week? What do you think 'damaged client' means in psychoanalytic terms? Do you agree with him that the process of change has to be inevitably slow?

I have worked with persons that were suffering from bulimia, who had been seeing psychoanalysts three, four or even five times a week for two to three years: they uncovered a lot of unconscious material and, at the same time, got deeper and deeper into their problem.

I have never thought of them as 'damaged' persons in their entirety, or as neurotic or deeply disturbed individuals. I have decided to focus on their healthy elements rather than on the ones in emergency functioning and have helped them through a person care approach involving approximately fifteen meetings, once a week (more or less the same model presented here in a step-by-step format).

They did stop vomiting, did stop bingeing and left the bulimic mind-set behind. This was almost four years ago and they are still in a great place now. What is this telling us? I am not a miracle worker and my person care model could not be simpler. This is exactly the point. Do we still need the outdated psychoanalytic paraphernalia to make sense of persons' issues and help them find the way out of their distress?

With all undue respect, I think that many psychoanalytic theories have clearly had their day. They never got anywhere near to the original philosophical Greek models, so dear to Freud, in the first place, and it is my personal opinion that continuing to apply them today, is, at best, a waste of time and of financial resources, a luxury for those who can afford weekly appointments with the hairdresser, the manicurist, the masseur, and the psychotherapist, and, at worst, potentially damaging to people's psychological health.

In many cases introspective therapy may encourage the person's tendency to over-analyse their life, thus pushing sufferers deeper into their distress without having lead them, first, to a safer place.

Freud himself recommended psychoanalysis to our interest 'not as a therapy, but rather because of what it reveals to us about what concerns man most closely: his own essence; and because of the connotations it uncovers between the widest variety of his actions.' (39)

There can also be no doubt that Freud viewed psychoanalysis as a truly humanistic undertaking, rather than a medical procedure or a cold and interpretative activity. He clearly stated that psychoanalysis was a *kulturarbeit*, which means, literally, "labour to achieve culture". (40)

I would like to think that Integrated Person Care has taken on board the true essence of Freud's inspiration by embracing the whole person (physiological, emotional, rational and behavioural components) without using medical or religious means of investigation or of interaction. IPC is not yet another form of psychotherapy: it is a *kulturarbeit*, an entirely human process of personal and cultural growth, where the person is warmly embraced with respect and attention and not considered as a *damaged* good.

Naturally, I have not created holism: holistic psychological approaches have been around since the times of Alfred Adler (he was born in 1870), who maintained that symptoms cannot be viewed in isolation from the whole person, who in turn cannot be viewed in isolation from the environment in which he or she lives. Each holistic model, however, has its own way of embracing the person, and IPC is no exception.

Likewise, the first attempts on the practitioners' part at giving up patronising the 'patient', and at starting, instead, from the sufferers' viewpoints to try to make sense of their issues, rather than moving from the practitioners' ones, as psychoanalysts do, can go back to Moreno's work in Vienna at the beginning of the 20th century (1913-1914).

Romanian born psychiatrist Jacob Moreno, moved first to Vienna and then to the US. He is the father of group psychotherapy and of psychodrama, whose first applications were tested in Vienna between 1913 and 1925.

A quantum leap forward in psychotherapy was made when cognitive therapy appeared on the scene, and I do agree with Beck when he says that 'man has the key to understanding and solving his psychological disturbance within the scope of his own awareness.' (41)

I also agree with him when he maintains that 'preliminary coaching of the patient about the type of therapy selected appears to enhance its effectiveness.' (42) However, I could not disagree more when he notes how 'Psychotherapy can have the greatest impact on problems because of the considerable authority attributed to the therapist, his ability to pinpoint the problems and his skill in providing an appropriate systematic set of procedures.' (43) I think he is placing the practitioner on too a high pedestal here, a bit far from view and from reality too!

I believe that what has the greatest impact on people's distress is genuine human sharing, and, in spite of the best efforts produced by some practitioners to shy away from that and maintain the distance between the person and them, psychotherapy still is a form of human interaction: that's why psychotherapy, despite the heavy shackles imposed by old (psychoanalysis) and new (cognitive behavioural therapy) masters, still manages to offer some help.

The key point is not the practitioners' interpretation of the person's issues and of how they think they would like to help, but, rather is the person's perception that they are helping themselves through the sharing of their problem with somebody whom they respect and trust not out of 'authority' but out of empathy and understanding.

An example of how the practitioners' skills and set of procedures can get in the way of the person's recovery process is offered by the following observations by Dr Bessel van der Kolk – a world famous expert in psychological trauma – on the treatment of post-traumatic stress disorders (PTSD):

"Experience shows that when people are asked to put their trauma into words, while they are in the process of re-living it, this can be enormously upsetting, and sometimes even impossible. Re-living the trauma without being firmly anchored in the here-and-now leaves people with PTSD often more traumatised than they were before.

Recalling the trauma can be so painful that many patients choose not to expose themselves to situations in which they are asked to do so, including to exposure therapies...So, when treating PTSD one central challenge is how to help people process and integrate their traumatic experiences without making them feel traumatized all over again, or, in the language of neuroscience: how to process trauma so that it is quenched, rather than re-kindled." (44)

IPC deals with the above challenge of helping people process and integrate their traumatic experiences without making them feel traumatised again, by avoiding the use of de-briefing and by focussing on the resetting of their systems, instead.

Once again, we favour a person care intervention to a psychotherapeutic one: the focus is not addressing the single event or its resulting symptoms, but helping the person, as a whole, through the resetting process, first, of the physiological component, and then, of the emotional and rational ones.

Then again, the above resetting can be done in many different ways.

Dr van der Kolk also notes elsewhere how:
"The imprint of trauma is the imprint on people's senses, on people's sensory systems. That becomes particularly important because these sensations stay in people's memory banks and stay unprocessed. If you do effective trauma processing, the individual smells, sounds, images and physical impressions of the trauma slowly disappear over time and that is something that doesn't happen with talking. It happens by working with people's bodily states. When a person experiences trauma, they become highly aroused and, for a period of time, lose their capacity for self-regulation. Parts of the frontal lobe that deal with the capacity to plan, to rationalise, to inhibit inappropriate behaviour – and specifically one area associated with speech – are shown to shut down. People who have experienced trauma need to feel safe in their bodies again. It's via the awareness of deep bodily experience that people can begin to move around the way they feel." (45)

In his view, this can be achieved by being still and noticing what is going on internally. A variety of gentle forms of exercise such as yoga, tai chi and dance, can allow this to happen and help the person feel and remain safe, grounded and embodied. That's why I have created Peaceflow: a new practice – introduced in my latest book, titled 'Peaceflow' – which integrates gentle bodywork and psychological techniques.

Arnold Lazarus, one of the most eminent exponents of the cognitive behaviour approach and the father of Multimodal Therapy – a brief and comprehensive model of intervention – notes how 'effective therapy depends far less on the hours you put in than in what you put in those hours' (46) and stresses the value of 'breadth over depth in therapy.' (47)

I do agree with him, and I share his view that a 'working alliance (Carl Rogers) is usually necessary but often insufficient', and that 'the more people learn in therapy, the less likely they are to relapse.' (48)

I also have the same opinion on the unhealthy language that most of us use on a daily basis. American psychologist Karen Horney was, to my knowledge, the first to clearly refer to 'the tyranny of the should' in 1950. Lazarus takes on board Horney's viewpoint by observing how 'the more categorical imperatives (should, must, have to) to which one subscribes the more anxious, hostile, guilt ridden and depressed one is likely to be.' (49)

However, I don't share Lazarus' view on the essential components of the psychological intervention. Multimodal Therapy is learning-based, problem-focused and solution-oriented. Integrated Person Care is learning-based, person-focused (we are more than our current issues) and process-oriented (life will keep on throwing challenges at us, learning and mastering the person care process is more important than focusing only on the solution to specific current problems).

I also find Lazarus' BASIC ID working model (Behaviour Affect Sensation Imagery Cognition Interpersonal Drugs-biology) a bit convoluted and artificial, as opposed to the more immediate and direct four components (physiological, emotional, rational and behavioural), three dimensions (intrapersonal, personal and interpersonal), and three time perspectives (past, present and future) of the IPC process.

Furthermore, while Lazarus views relaxation methods simply as 'sensory techniques' (50), IPC attributes to the practice of relaxation a central psychological value.

I have already acknowledged Albert Ellis' contribution to applied psychology, but, just changing the name of his approach – from Rational Therapy to Rational Emotive Therapy, as he did in 1961, before changing it again to Rational Emotive Behaviour Therapy in 1993 – does not change the basic and crystal clear facts that irrational beliefs are seen as the cause of emotional and behavioural problems and that emotions are only mentioned when the practitioner and the person are strongly encouraged to reconsider them in the light of rational thinking.

As Albert Ellis observes: *"Keep forcefully and persistently disputing your irrational beliefs whenever you see that you are letting them creep back again. And even when you don't actively hold them, realize that they may arise once more, bring them to your consciousness, and preventively – and vigorously! – dispute them…Convincing yourself lightly or 'intellectually' of your new effective philosophy or rational beliefs often won't help very much or persist very long. Do so very strongly and vigorously, and do so many times. Thus, you can powerfully convince yourself, until you really feel it…" (51)*

I believe that staging a fight between our rational and emotional components, where we ask our rational mind to *forcefully* and *vigorously* win by *convincing* our emotional self of its inadequacies, does not only fail to provide a long term truce to the dispute in place, but, it might reinforce the very behaviour it wants to eliminate: the 'all or nothing' unhealthy thinking style.

IPC, to the contrary, believes in the benefits of reconciling our different components: the answer is to show the person – who is into emergency functioning mode, rather than being overwhelmed by irrational beliefs – how to make peace with and within themselves.

I do believe that the most appropriate way to deal with an enemy – whether they be internal or external – is to make peace with them: only a just peace involving and accommodating all the parties in question (physiological, emotional, rational and behavioural components) can guarantee a long term resolution to our psychological distress.

Moreover, REBT does not offer any direct indication of how to address our emotional selves and, most importantly, holds the belief that we can change the way we feel by changing the way we think.

As already mentioned, the latest research development in neuroscience appears to have shown that, when we think, we use and relate only to our rational brain and we do not get through, by means of mere logical thinking, to our emotional selves.

I completely agree, then, with Robert Lefever when he notes:

"... even psychological treatments can be misguided. Currently the form of psychotherapy favoured by most doctors tends to be cognitive-behavioural. In this approach the doctor or therapist calmly explains to the patient what he or she has misconceived and tells him or her, what would be better. It sounds sensible and it flatters doctors and therapists who think that they always know the answers. However, for exactly those reasons, it can be patronising and ultimately totally ineffectual. One cannot treat an irrational problem with reason: it would not be an irrational problem if one could." (52)

In total agreement with what is stated above, IPC practitioners don't provide *answers* to the persons in their care: they share an inter-existential space – that is, a place and a time where the practitioner can stimulate the person's connection with their life forces by *simply* being there and by presenting a clear, practical, person care process.

The IPC practitioner – unlike CBT or NLP practitioners – does not *correct* or *restructure* the person's thinking by imposing models which are completely alien, both to their experience and the way of perceiving themselves and the world. Sooner, rather than later, the person will disassociate from CBT reframing and NLP techniques, because they don't belong to their real life: their daily life experience reflects their own uniqueness, which cannot be matched by models originated some thirty or fifty years ago by somebody living in another continent.

The IPC process, instead, helps the person connect with their *own* capacity for change and growth – a deeper awareness which nothing and nobody will be able to take away from them. Only the person has the power to disconnect from them. Only the person has the power to reconnect with their own life forces and inner wisdom.

Without the capacity of regenerating themselves no living organism on this planet would survive: human beings are the zenith of evolution on Earth and each of the billions of cells which make up who we are possess this capacity for regeneration.

We have the choice. We can connect with these enormously powerful life forces and address our current distress now by choosing a person care path, or we keep on playing someone else's mind games until our next relapse into stress and depression, by opting for outdated models and techniques.

One of the questions I am often asked is: "What is the difference between the Integrated Person Care view of the human system and the psychosomatic one?"

Very simply put, the psychosomatic approach maintains that our psychological distress may **cause** our physical discomfort, and our physical discomfort may **cause** psychological distress: we are, therefore, in the presence of a circular cause-effect dynamic.

IPC views, instead, the human being as a unitary system where there is no causal link between mind and body: there is only one mindbodyspirit entity. Due to the limitation of their senses, humans can only perceive and approach this wonderfully integrated system partially and selectively.

Therefore, when in IPC we refer to 'mind', 'body', 'components', 'selves', we do so only for the sake of simplicity, because of the way we make sense of our reality.

Human beings cannot comprehend and classify their creator: a person cannot embrace or *understand* the totality of the mindbodyspirit system which creates them, every day.

Mindful of the above, in IPC we help the person reconnect with their own vital resources gently and gradually: always respecting and supporting the person's uniqueness and the different ways in which they selectively view themselves and the world.

Activities Box 9.

Time for your *PAL* …
Briefly summarise the differences between the psychoanalytic, cognitive and integrated person care models.

and for your *BIT.*
Write down your negative thoughts as soon as you are aware of them and observe your physical and emotional response to them.

Therapeutic relationship or person care process?

Practitioners, who see patients or clients in sessions where a psychotherapeutic model is applied, would define this interaction as the 'therapeutic relationship'. Practitioners, who get together with persons in meeting where the Integrated Person Care approach is embraced, would refer to this interpersonal experience simply as the 'person care process'.

IPC practitioners aim at making their support redundant, as soon as this is appropriate. Some practitioners do not object to enjoying the incomes coming from very long term 'therapeutic relationships' with their patients. I believe that the accustoming of the person to the practitioner becomes, in the long run, a form of addiction and, as such, it ends up dispensing more harm than benefits – apart from the obvious doubts arising on the effectiveness of such lengthy 'treatments' or 'analyses', that is.

Psychoanalytic practitioners can carry on seeing a person forever, because exploring their patients' whys is a never-ending mind game. The professional experience of practitioners adopting different models (i.e. behavioural or cognitive) over the past fifty years has clearly shown that it is possible to help people out of their distress without fully investigating their whys, by focussing instead on *what* is happening to them and *how* to overcome their current situation.

I am not saying here that those who undergo a long process of analytic therapy never find it useful or get better. I am saying that in those cases when they do find it useful and feel better, this happens in spite of, rather than thanks to, the approach used. In other words, in such cases the practitioner's personal qualities and the long-term human interaction between them and their patients manage to provide a basic relief that the adopted model does not even contemplate.

IPC acknowledges that most people have within themselves (or within their reach) the resources they require to face and overcome their personal distress: all they may call for, when they find it difficult to do this on their own, is a little help to reset their system and start up the recovery process. The practitioner, therefore, is there only to provide this help and to support the person back to their social reality (i.e. friends and family).

The aim is to comfortably and steadily let the macrocosm of the persons' daily life experiences replace the microcosm of the meeting occurring in the practitioner's consulting room, allowing the practitioner and their supporting role to discretely fade away.

Activities Box 10.

Time for your *PAL* ...
Did you know that it is possible to help somebody out of their distress without getting deep into their whys? If you did, what were your first thoughts when you learnt about it? If you didn't, what are your thoughts now?

and for your *BIT*.
Write down your positive thoughts as soon as you are aware of them and observe your physical and emotional response to them.

Chapter 4

Practising IPC

"A neurotic is a man who builds a castle in the air.
A psychotic is the man who lives in it.
A psychiatrist is the man who collects the rent."

Jerome Lawrence (1)

Do we need professional help?

Many try to 'sort themselves out' on their own and that is perfectly acceptable: we can do a pretty good job on our own. However, others may not feel able or ready, as yet, to work on their issues by themselves and, at the same time, still feel wary about seeking professional help.

This could be because of what they have heard or read about some practitioners, because they confuse psychology or counselling with psychiatry ('I am not mad, why should I talk to a shrink?'), because they think that all practitioners practise in a psychoanalytic way ('What's the point in talking about my father and my childhood, when my problem is that jerk of a manager that I face everyday at work?'), or because they do not have the financial means to fund their meetings with a private practitioner and they prefer to stay away from the services provided by the National Health Service because they don't want their issues filed in medical records.

If we consider that we are not dealing here with severe mental health problems but, rather, with problems that, at one time or another, may affect any of us, we might wonder if we do really need to seek help from a psychological practitioner or if we would be better off taking care of our issues either by ourselves, or with the help of a friend or relative.

I think that friends and relatives can provide valuable help. However, whichever way we look at it, they are very much part of our life and what we say to them, or do with them, will sooner or later come back to us, in one form or another.

Because of their emotional involvement with us, a close friend or relative is not in a position to offer any of the following:

59

- *aporein*, the old Greek for 'doubt', that is the capacity to see you as a new person, and, as such, to relate to you with an open mind, ready and able to exercise the art of doubting what you say or do;

- *epoche*`, the old Greek for 'suspension of judgement', that is to be in a position of not having any interest whatsoever in your personal choices, whichever direction you decide to pursue;

- *apatheia*, the old Greek for 'detachment from passions', that is to be able to connect with you without necessarily sharing your emotional states or rational concerns.

In my view, therefore, the real point is not *whether* we would benefit from professional help, but, rather, *what* type of help would be most appropriate, given our personal circumstances.

I believe that we *can* help ourselves by choosing a clear path towards recovery and by working gradually and surely towards the new person we would like to become. We can do this either by following a step-by-step programme, which can be found in a useful self-help book (like I hope this one will turn out to be for you!), or by choosing a suitable practitioner, or by a combination of the two.

What I would like to provide you with, in the next sections of this chapter, is a brief and clear indication of what is on offer out there, in terms of available professional help.

I will, first, discuss the issue of taking medication. Then, I will introduce you to the main psychological disciplines dealing with personal distress and I will offer a clarification of the main approaches being applied today and of the way individual practitioners may differ from one another. Finally, I will present a brief overview of the
steps that make up the Integrated Person Care model.

Activities Box 11.

Time for your *PAL* ...
Think about the persons (i.e. close friends, relatives) you know you can count on to help you deal with your current problems. Note down their names.

and for your *BIT.*
Get in touch, anyway you prefer (i.e. by phone, letter or by email) with one or two of the persons above and let them know that you have decided to work on your issues by following the step-by-step approach of this guide. Ask if they are willing to be there for you, in case you need to talk or to meet with them, and agree mutually convenient times and means of staying in touch (email correspondence would do). From now on we will refer to this person(s) as your 'travel mate'.

Do we need antidepressants?

One of the common questions I am asked in the consulting room is whether I recommend the use of antidepressants, or rely entirely on my person care process. In that setting I normally provide the following short answer: 'I will not encourage you to take antidepressants. However, if you are already on medication do not discontinue your treatment at this stage and, as you will progress through your person care process, you may agree with your medical practitioner how and when to gradually phase out your medication.'

Here, I would like to provide a slightly more articulated answer to the above question. First, I will offer the views of well-respected professionals and, then, I will present my own reflections.

Jerome Burne points out how:
"New Scientist ran an article on the new view of depression that suggests a key factor is damage to the neurons in a part of the emotional brain known as the hippocampus, involved with memory and learning. This damage seems to be linked with excess amounts of the stress hormone cortisol.

This new view means that the one theory about depression that everyone is familiar with – that is linked with low serotonin levels – is almost certainly wrong. Instead, the spotlight is on another brain chemical called BDNF (brain-derived neurotrophic factor) that helps cells in the hippocampus regrow. The article enthused about a new generation of antidepressants that this could lead to. What it didn't emphasise was that drugs aren't the only way to raise BDNF levels. Exercise, omega-3 oils (which can be found in oily fish such as herring, salmon, mackerel and sardines, olive oil, and walnuts) and acupuncture can do it as well." (2)

British psychiatrist David Healy notes: "...depression is a disorder of the whole person, existential or social distress marked by unhappiness and hopelessness. It is cast into physical symptoms precisely because they have been made fashionable, sanctioned and publicised by today's medical-industrial complex." (3)

In reviewing one of Healy's publications, professor Canter observes:
"It used to be all repressed urges or childhood abuse. Now, the root cause of sadness is low levels of serotonin. Psychobabble has given way to biobabble. And as psychotropic drugs to treat the levels of feel-good brain chemicals proliferate, the definitions of all kinds of mental suffering are changing... Everyone from psychopaths, drug abusers and paedophiles to the shy and unhappy are all now seen as manageable through pills and potions. Healy uncovers the interrelated mix of forces that have driven us to look to drugs as the answer to these psychological and social discomforts. The interests of the pharmaceuticals industry itself are not the least of these forces. As Healy says, the industry "has highly developed capacities to gather and market evidence favourable to its business interests". Healy shows how this, combined with the political interests of medicine, has created flawed procedures that are then used to defend the power of drugs. These include misdiagnoses, crude qualitative models of mental illness rather than more complex multidimensional ones, and evaluation procedures that rely on artificially controlled conditions rather than direct clinical experience." (4)

Why is this happening? What are the reasons behind the rise in the use of antidepressants? As professor Small points out, there could be a few million good reasons:
"As well as being a threat to health, depression is hugely expensive. Medication is the treatment favoured by doctors and patients alike: over 22 million prescriptions were written for antidepressants in England in 2000, a rise of a third in only 10 years. In Britain, as a whole, the bill for these drugs stands at

£296 million a year, while the cost associated with loss of production and invalidity benefits is as high as £8 billion each year." (5)

So, is this all about money? I don't think so. Are doctors aware of what's going on? Of course, they are. Dr Robert Lefever, a medical practitioner with many years of practice under his belt, notes:
"Patients need to be helped towards feeling the full range of their emotions and learning to react appropriately so that they have a full and stimulating life. The alternative of suppressing their feelings with sugar and white flour or with the mood-altering effects of bingeing, starving, vomiting or purging, leads to a drab and colourless existence. Great claims are often made for what is achieved through taking antidepressants. The real tragedy of their widespread use is in observing what is taken away: the spontaneity, creativity and enthusiasm that are the essence of life itself...Furthermore, variation of mood is precisely what gives life its colour and to homogenise it with antidepressants is a terrible thing to do to people. A life without colour may be functional but it has surely lost much of its value." (6)

So, if it is not about money, why is this state of affairs carrying on? If we want to look and see, the answer is there before our eyes. When people consult their doctor and are prescribed their medication everyone is happy, because they all go down the easiest path.

Persons, now turned into *patients,* are happy because rather than facing up to their problems and having to introduce changes in their lives, are now simply required to take a pill once or twice a day. I have seen many persons that really wanted to be diagnosed with some sort of disorder – though there was no indication of any – just because they were looking for an easy way out, rather than taking their life's difficult turn as an opportunity to grow up.

Medical practitioners, now turned into prescription-dispensers, are happy because there's not much else they can do in a 10 minutes' consultation. After all, they are medically trained professionals not policy makers and they are to abide by the rules, as the rest of us. What's the point in referring somebody to a psychological practitioner when there is a five to ten months' waiting list?

Governments, now admirably turned into money-saving organisations, are happy because pills cost far less than psychological interventions and, above all, are more straightforward, easy to apply and politically correct than the implementation of proper health care initiatives at the personal and social level.

Finally, pharmaceutical companies are very happy, indeed, because profits margins are huge in this line of business.

I certainly believe that, in the presence of severe mental illnesses, the use of medication can benefit both the sufferers and their families – though, when it comes to dealing with anti-social behaviour, there can be no substitute to the care provided by an appropriately supervised setting. However, it looks like prescriptions of antidepressants have now reached such a level that I would warmly encourage those who are experiencing personal distress to reconsider their approach to their problems and their feelings of unhappiness.

Working on our issues is not as easy as taking a pill, but it is much more rewarding and, in the end, the only true way out of them.

Activities Box 12.

Time for your *PAL* …
Have you ever taken medication? What's your view on antidepressants?

and for your *BIT*.
Ask somebody whom you know well, or your travel mate, if they have taken antidepressants and what's their view on them?

Main disciplines dealing with personal distress.

Before the conception of Integrated Person Care in the summer of 1991, and its first applications, psychological distress has been dealt with by one of the following disciplines.

Counselling and Psychotherapy.
Often termed 'talking therapies' they might also involve other forms of creative expression such as art, drama, music, dance or play. Some people use the terms counselling and psychotherapy interchangeably, others, from well-established traditions (i.e. psychoanalytic psychotherapy), distinguish between them.
Counselling is a form of psychological therapy that gives individuals an opportunity to explore, discover and clarify ways of living more resourcefully, with a greater sense of well being.

Counsellors may adopt a specific model or a combination of approaches (i.e. humanistic, psychodynamic, cognitive-behavioural). Counsellors may start practising under supervision following completion of a Foundation course and of a primary course in their chosen approach. To become a qualified counsellor you are mainly required to have practised under supervision for a minimum of three years, have undertaken a certain amount of training hours – which vary according to the accreditation route chosen – and to commit to personal and professional development.

The main professional body for counsellors in the UK is the British Association for Counselling and Psychotherapy (BACP).

Psychotherapy is a form of psychological therapy that intends to relieve or heal a disorder. Psychotherapists may practise within any or a combination of approaches (i.e. psychoanalysis, gestalt, cognitive-behavioural) and the beginning of their practice depends on the chosen model.

To become a qualified psychotherapist you are mainly required to have practised under supervision for a minimum of three to four years, have undertaken a certain amount of training hours – which vary according to the accreditation route chosen – and to commit to personal and professional development.

The main professional bodies for psychotherapists in the UK are the British Association for Counselling and Psychotherapy (BACP) and the United Kingdom Council for Psychotherapy (UKCP).

Counselling and Clinical Psychology.

Counselling Psychology applies psychology to working collaboratively across a diverse range of human problems. These include helping people manage difficult life events such as bereavement, past and present relationships and working with mental issues and disorders. Counselling psychologists explore underlying issues and use an active collaborative relationship to empower people to consider change.

Clinical Psychology aims to reduce psychological distress and to enhance and promote psychological well being. Psychological difficulties that are dealt with include anxiety, depression, learning disabilities and serious mental illness.

Generally, a clinical psychologist undertakes a clinical assessment which may lead to therapy, counselling or advice.

The professional body for psychologists in the UK is the British Psychological Society (BPS). To practice as a Counselling or as a Clinical Psychologist you are required, first, to hold a first degree which grants you the Graduate Basis for Registration (GBR) with the BPS, and, then, to undertake a three-year postgraduate training.

Psychiatry.

Psychiatry studies and treats mental diseases, such as disorders in childhood and adolescence, psychoses including schizophrenia, mania, bipolar disorders and organic brain syndromes.

Psychiatrists may use either pharmacological therapy, psychotherapy or a combination of both. When they adopt psychotherapeutic interventions, they apply any or a combination of the main approaches indicated above.

To become a psychiatrist you are first required to undertake medical studies and training, and, then, to specialise in psychiatry. The professional body for psychiatrists in the UK is the Royal College of Psychiatrists.

Coaching.

Coaching is the teaching of skills aimed at improving competency in a generic (i.e. life coaching) or a specific (i.e. fear of flying) area. By definition, coaching is present and future oriented: past issues or traumas are not addressed by means of skills' training. There is a variety of coaching training programmes on offer as well as a number of professional associations. As a first point of reference in the UK you may contact the Association for Coaching.

Now that you know a bit more about the main disciplines addressing psychological issues, let's take a look at what really counts, when it comes to receiving professional help.

Activities Box 13.

Time for your *PAL* ...
What are the most important factors you are likely to consider, when choosing a psychological practitioner?

and for your *BIT.*
Browse through the websites of the BACP, the BPS and the School of Integrated Person Care (see addresses in the resources section of this guide). What is the first feeling that you get when you access them and how helpful do you find them?

Talking therapies.

When it comes to psychological help – commonly referred to as 'talking therapy' – you will find yourself puzzled by a number of different options.

The choice of a practitioner is surely an important one. As David Smail notes: "...many studies have shown that, at least for the 'talking therapies' ... what counts most towards patients' recovery is precisely not the theoretical inclinations of the practitioners, but their personality, i.e. how far patients feel able to talk to them and to trust them, how likeable they find them." (7)

Now, I believe that finding ourselves at ease with a practitioner is an essential but not a sufficient condition, if we want to address successfully our issues.

In other words, I think that it is well worth considering not only if we find ourselves comfortable – on a human level – with a practitioner, but, also, if we and our distress 'fit in' with their working model.

You would not walk into a florist if you were hungry and looking for food, and if you did walk in by mistake, you would not eat their flowers, no matter how nice and polite the florists were! Well, as odd as this might seem, the truth is that many of us 'do eat the flowers', as we end up seeing a practitioner just because they are nice and without having a clue of what their approach is, or of what their therapeutic model implies, or of how their way of working could eventually help prevent or overcome our distress.

So, we might end up seeing an analyst three times a week for two years to no avail, for a problem which could have been properly addressed by means of a 15-session programme. To the contrary, we might feel disillusioned and let down when our issues have not been appropriately dealt with through a brief intervention and a medium term approach would have been more beneficial.

So, how do we know? Well, this is precisely one of my points. I believe that each and every practitioner has a duty to offer to the person looking for help and support, at the earliest possible stage (i.e. first phone conversation or initial consultation) the following information, by brief oral communication or by means of printed materials (i.e. leaflets, handouts):

⇒ clear indication of their working model;
⇒ main characteristics and objectives of their approach;
⇒ pros and cons, particularly with regard to the person's presenting issues;

$\Rightarrow$ indication of how other approaches may address their problems, or referrals to relevant sources, which can provide further information (i.e. useful websites of professional bodies).

I appreciate, however, that it could be very difficult to receive a certain level of service, if you don't know that you have a right to demand that standard of care.

Therefore, the second important point I am making here is: know your rights, ask questions and make sure that you are entirely satisfied both with your chosen practitioner and their approach, before you start working with them.

I could not agree more with David Smail when he says that "ordinary people are perfectly capable of expressing and understanding any theory about their problems you care to name...and can detect intellectual and professional bullshit a mile off." (8)

So, to help you make an informed decision, the next paragraph will offer a brief illustration of the three main approaches to personal distress together with concise explanatory notes about Integrated Person Care.

Activities Box 14.

Time for your *PAL* ...
Which one of the following labels sounds appropriate to you, when it comes to name somebody who is seeing a psychological practitioner: patient, client or person?

and for your *BIT*.
Discuss the above with your travel mate.

Common approaches and IPC.

As you read through, please bear in mind that different approaches work differently for different people. In other words, the point is not which one is right or which one is wrong, in absolute terms, but, rather, which one you feel and think would best suit both you and your personal issues.

Psychoanalysis.

The analytic practitioner will listen to you and will help you bring to the surface deeply buried unconscious material, attempting, in so doing, to clarify the connections between past events and present distress. It usually involves long term work (a year or more) and between one and five sessions a week. It can help you get to know yourself better and get to your 'whys', but the therapist will never offer you directions (i.e. 'how' to overcome your problems).

On a practical level, you may end up seeing an analyst for years without introducing a single change in your life. So, if you are the kind of person that would love to indulge in long talks with an intelligent listener or if you relish the thought of engaging in deeply sophisticated mind games, analysis is definitely for you!

Your analyst will never push you into any direction and you may see them for as long as you wish: some see the same analyst for ten or fifteen years, or more.

IPC does acknowledge the importance of past events, so much so that our preliminary work, the 'opening stage', is concerned with the exploration of emotional issues and rational processes. However, in IPC, this stage only takes five meetings to help you focus precious time, energy and motivation on the creation of the person you would like to become.

Humanistic Counselling.

A number of very different schools (i.e. Rogerian person-centred, Gestalt) share nonetheless a set of common 'humanistic' values. The practitioner will use a warmer approach than the analytic/interpretative one. You will be encouraged to express yourself and to reflect on your problems. The emphasis here is on your present strengths and future possibilities: your potential for positive change. The practitioner will not give you advice as to how to prevent and overcome your issues, directly, but you will be helped to find them on your own.

IPC shares the above humanistic values and, at the same time, takes two further considerable steps:

a) You will have the opportunity not only to explore your inner world and to communicate your feelings, but you will also share with the practitioner 'how' you relate to the 'all' of yourself (physiological, emotional and rational components) and you will receive valuable feedback and information not just on 'what' to do, but on 'how' to take care of yourself.

b) Our programme is not just about listening and counselling, it is also about teaching and training. The practitioner will pass on to you a number of skills and techniques, which will be relevant to your distress.

Cognitive Behaviour Therapies.

Cognitive practitioners believe that by changing ('reframing') our thought processes we can change how we feel and what we do. Behavioural practitioners, on the other hand, maintain that by changing our behaviour we can, then, change how we feel and what we think. Time, practical wisdom and necessity have brought these two approaches together and cognitive behaviour therapy (CBT) is very fashionable today. A number of different CBTs are currently being practised (i.e. Beck's cognitive therapy, Ellis' rational emotive behavioural therapy, Lazarus' multimodal therapy). The practitioners will help you change those patterns of negative thinking or self-defeating behaviour that are causing problems. They will agree goals for treatment with you and you will practise the new skills learnt in your own time between sessions.

As we have seen above, empowering you – by providing training in emotional and rational management – is one of the activities carried out in our person care programme. IPC also shares with CBT approaches recognition of the usefulness of working towards the person's recovery in a clear and focussed way. However, IPC does something more for you:

a) From the very first meeting, and throughout the whole of our person care process, the basic counselling element is always there. This means that a practitioner practising IPC will treat you as a person, will connect with you and take your emotional issues into account. One of the common complaints I receive by persons, who come to me after having run away from an orthodox CBT practitioner, is that they were rigidly following their scripts, without any acknowledgement whatsoever of the person's current emotional situation. To the contrary, we do take time to help you explore your emotional level and to help you understand and connect with your emotional states.

b) In CBT persons are often too quickly diagnosed, labelled and sent through a pre-determined and structured programme where their negative thinking is reframed and their self-defeating behaviour is challenged. In IPC, to the contrary, you will be first guided through a journey of self-discovery and taught how to reconnect with your own body and with your emotional and rational components; then, you will learn how to re-associate with your intrapersonal, personal and interpersonal dimensions and you will reconsider your approach to the three time perspectives: past, present and future. The person's input here is far greater than the one allowed by CBT, and, not surprisingly, persons feel much more comfortable when going through the IPC process, and this, in turn, greatly helps them through their journey of recovery.

c) Persons are allowed to go through the above process at their own pace: some find it appropriate to meet once a week, whereas others find it useful to work intensively on their issues (i.e. 2 or 3 hour, or half-day, meetings).

The above person care process can be effective without requiring a long term intervention. IPC believes in the benefits of intensive and focussed work, as demonstrated by a number of intensive interventions, which have been successfully delivered since January 2000.

Positive psychology.

Founded in 1998 by American psychologist, Martin Seligman, the positive psychology movement 'focuses on cultivating personality strengths and honing an optimistic approach to life rather than on cataloguing human frailty and disease'. (9) Seligman says 'After 60 years, clinical psychology can claim that it makes miserable people less miserable, but what about the person who wants to go from a plus three to a plus eight?'

To do that, positive psychologists ask persons to carry out a series of exercises, such as:

- *the gratitude letter,* where you are asked to pick a person in your life whom you would like to thank, someone who has meant a lot to you, and write this person a letter;

- *the gratitude visit,* where you may call the person you have written the letter, ask to visit and, once there, read the letter aloud to them;

71

□ *the strengths test,* where you are asked to choose and score your good personality traits (i.e. wisdom or love), which are in turn divided into strengths (i.e. love is broken down into intimacy, kindness and social intelligence).

Seligman believes that knowing your strengths makes it easier to achieve more meaningful forms of happiness. As Willow Lawson notes: "Seligman's blend of self-awareness and optimistic thinking is hardly new, but novelty is not a selling point: Seligman freely admits that he draws on a large body of research from Mihaly Csikszentmihalyi's concept of 'flow', or absorption in a task, to Robert Emmons' findings on gratitude. Positive psychologists are, however, the first group to pull together these strands, push for more research and zealously disseminate the results." (10)

IPC welcomes positive psychology, as you would welcome a breath of fresh air in the midst of a hot summer night. We share its emphasis on the dissemination of helpful and useful practical knowledge and its critique of orthodox clinical psychology. However, in real life, persons do not seek professional help because they want to get from 'plus three to plus eight': they come to us when they are down to minus seven or ten!

We, also, think that this would be a very sad world, if there was no room and space for sadness. Sadness has a value, like happiness, and IPC teaches how to achieve an appropriate balance between the two.

Prevention is better than cure.

While other approaches intervene only when your issues have become current, IPC believes in the value of preventative work and teaches practical techniques to help you prevent many forms of personal distress. Four centuries before Christ, the Sou wen – traditional manual of Chinese medicine – read: "Good doctors do not treat the sick, they teach the healthy. Curing a disease is like digging a well when you are thirsty, or like forging a sword when the battle has already begun." (11)

'Prevention is better than cure' is a motto which, in our western world, is as well-known as it is gloriously ignored, and even when it is put into practice, its application is rigorously confined to the realm of the physical body.

Why are we waiting for a traumatic event to happen to spring out of our boxes and try to put a smile on a distressed face? Wouldn't it be more appropriate to teach useful concepts and techniques before it is our turn to 'suffer from the slings and arrows' that life throws at us? Wouldn't it be wise learning emotional management and helpful thinking at a time when we are fully able to focus on what we are being taught because we are not experiencing the depth of psychological distress?

Conclusion.

IPC is a truly integrated model which:

1. integrates some important features of consolidated models such as Jungian analysis, humanistic counselling, cognitive therapy and behavioural techniques;

2. works through the entire person by addressing their physical, emotional, rational and behavioural components; their three dimensions (intrapersonal, personal and interpersonal) and time perspectives (past, present and future);

3. integrates Eastern wisdom with Western knowledge;

4. can be delivered 'traditionally' in weekly one-hour sessions, or intensively, for three hours or half-days;

5. has a clear and productive emphasis on preventative work;

6. is a versatile, step-by-step approach which is very practical and easy to apply.

7. integrates traditional verbal work with a new gentle bodywork practice, which I have created and called Peaceflow;

IPC regards the person care process as a truly personal and cultural achievement, rather than as a form of therapy. Integrated practitioners do not see 'patients' (a term that implies adherence to the medical-pathological perspective), or 'clients' (a term that evokes inter-dependency and consumerism), they work with 'persons'. Why use or refer to words that apply artificial layers onto who we are? We are, first and foremost, persons, and

Integrated Person Care is a process involving two persons: one who, just to avoid confusion, we call the *practitioner* and the other, who, therefore, we can simply call the *person*.

Activities Box 15.

Time for your *PAL* ...
When you think of short, medium or long-term programmes of psychological help, how many meetings would you associate with each of them?

and for your *BIT*.
Ask your travel mate the same question and discuss the resulting estimates with them.

Overview of the IPC process.

You will find here below a summary of the Integrated Person Care process, which will be presented, step by step, in the next chapters. Please note that one step does not correspond to one meeting: a single step may require two or more meetings or two steps can be addressed in just one meeting, depending on the person's background, life experience and presenting issues.

Some would like to proceed at a lower pace, while others at a faster one. There is, also, no need for a person to go through the entire programme: some may find it beneficial enough just to go through the its main components.

I have been able to carry out some good work with a minimum of 10 meetings.

As you can appreciate that does not depend on an alleged ability or expertise on my part, but, rather on the person's motivation to fully engage in the person care process and on the presenting problems.

Opening Stage:

Initial consultation
Lifestyle questionnaire
Emotional exploration (optional)
Rational exploration (optional)
Discussion

Resourcing stage:

Sensations
Behaviours
Emotions
Thoughts
Dimensions & Perspectives

Activities Box 16.

Time for your *PAL* …
Look back and reflect on what you have read so far.

and for your *BIT. Discuss the above with your travel mate.*

PART TWO

~

THE PERSON CARE PROCESS

~

Chapter 5
The Opening Stage

"What really counts it's not what you see:
it's that you are looking."

Gide (1)

Introducing the opening stage.

This part of the Integrated Person Care process is entirely optional. It is the IPC equivalent of a physical check-up and requires a practitioner to be carried out. Those who have time and money to invest in this exploration, may take an opportunity to get to know themselves better. Persons tend to find this stage very interesting and some have even felt that something had *clicked* during the emotional or the rational exploration. In a couple of occasions, I have had persons, who – despite having already pre-paid subsequent meetings – felt in such a different place from where they were before that they thanked me and never came back. At the same time, I have successfully carried out many person care processes by skipping the opening stage and starting straightaway from the resourcing stage.

The metaphor I normally use, when I explain to persons the difference between going through the opening stage and starting immediately from the resourcing stage, is that of somebody wanting to buy a suit. You may visit a tailor and have a made-to-measure garment or you can walk into a nice shop and choose the one you like: the first option will allow you a bit more of an insight into what you will be wearing, but either way you are a winner!

If you are a sufferer or a carer, you are advised to skip to the next chapter now and, if you wish, you may come back and read this chapter later. Please do not try and practise this stage with the help of a friend or relative: the emotional and rational explorations can get you to places where you would require the help of a trained practitioner for the journey back. If you are a qualified or trainee practitioner, please do carry on reading.

As I have already mentioned, I do not believe in quick psychological diagnoses and personality inventories.

When persons come and see me, that means that they are already in emergency functioning with one or more of their sensors going off. Therefore, I don't make any attempt at trying to understand their distress from my viewpoint. What I offer them, during the opening stage, is an opportunity to experience a brief but meaningful journey of guided exploration of their emotional issues and rational concerns.

In other words, I give them the chance to tell their story in many different ways (oral conversation, body language, lifestyle questionnaire, emotional and rational explorations) which are then openly discussed during the last meeting of this stage. This work can benefit the person care process, because I will know more about them and they will have had the chance to break the ice and test me, as their chosen guide.

I think that the process of recovery from personal distress will not even start if persons do not feel comfortable with their practitioners. That is why I regularly share moments of intense emotional pain when I hear how some practitioners may have had five or six meetings with a person without even looking at them once in their eyes! All caught up in their note-taking and graph-drawing activities, they do not care to ask a simple 'how are you?' That makes me wonder, what is clinical psychology, psychotherapy or psychiatry all about, if we do not even care to acknowledge the person's basic feelings?

I am not criticising fellow practitioners here. I am genuinely convinced that these professionals would not be working in their prestigious public or private settings if they were not more than experienced and qualified. But this is exactly the point. What is the use of years of education, training and continuing professional development, when our chosen working model leads us to gloriously ignore the person in front of us, the very reason we are there in that moment in time?

Are we there to help persons out of their distress or is our work about gaining validation for how clever and skilled we are? Aren't we confusing who is the protagonist and who is playing the supporting role here?

Aren't we forgetting that these are real persons and real life cases we are dealing with and not some statistical items to be entered in a research database and discussed at some point in a target-setting exercise or conference?

Activities Box 17.

Initial consultation.

The first meeting serves the following purposes:

- it gives an opportunity to both the practitioner and the person to see how they interact face-to-face;
- it allows the person to introduce their issues;
- it provides the appropriate time and place to let the practitioner present the kinds of psychological help on offer as well as their chosen approach;
- it offers the person the chance to have some of their questions answered by the practitioner.

In order to meet the above goals, I normally divide my 60-minute initial consultations into four parts:

The first part (20 minutes) is dedicated to the persons' introduction of their problems. I start by presenting how I usually use the 60 minutes of the first meeting and ask the person if they are happy to follow this format.

Then, I invite them to talk and I rarely interrupt the flow of their recollections reserving any question I might wish to ask to the second part. It is quite useful to agree from the start how the time will be used: this way the person will not feel disregarded when you note that it's time to move on to the next part of the meeting. This will also help you keep your time-boundary and, most importantly, will allow you to meet all of the main goals of the first meeting.

I use the second part (10 minutes) to ask the person what are their expectations of the psychological process. My standard question is 'if you didn't mind my Italian accent and you found my approach suitable, what would you like to achieve at the end of our programme, where would you like me to take you?'

I fully appreciate that persons are still in 'emergency functioning' at this stage, so this question is not meant to introduce a goal-setting activity. What I look for here is a basic appreciation of the person's expectations, to help me find out if I am the right practitioner for them.

The sooner we realise we are not equipped to deal with a specific issue, the sooner it would be appropriate to refer the person on by providing them with as much relevant information as we can.

So, for example, if a lady were to answer 'I am getting married in 8 weeks and would like to lose 2 stones', I would tell her that I do not specialise in crash diets, that I would not recommend one – as we know how unhealthy they can be – and I would refer her to a dietician.

The third part (15 minutes) allows the practitioner the opportunity to briefly present the main psychological approaches and their own orientation. I normally spend ten minutes presenting pros and cons of the analytical, humanistic and cognitive-behavioural models and then I leave the remaining five minutes for a concise illustration of the IPC model.

As you can appreciate, there is not much you can get across in 15 minutes and that's why I hand over to them some literature on the above topics (i.e. leaflets, my website address, copy of my person care contract, etc.).

During the fourth and final part (15 minutes) persons are free to ask any question they may wish. I always take care of reminding them that what is really important is not whether they decide to start working through their issues with me or not, but, rather, that they don't lose the motivation to address them.

Therefore, I invite them to call me, or to drop me an email, and to ask me anything that did not cross their mind during our initial consultation. In other words, I ask them to see me as a resource, whether they would like to carry on with me or not, because when the latter applies, I would be happy to provide them with further useful information.

Activities Box 18.

Lifestyle questionnaire.

Sometimes persons provide me – prior to our initial consultation or during it – with a letter, which includes details about the history of their issue as well as relevant additional information (i.e. family and professional backgrounds). However, in most cases they don't, so I ask them to fill in – in their own time at home – a lifestyle questionnaire. I normally read questionnaires in my own time – usually on Friday mornings, when I prepare for the meetings I will be having during the following week.

I do not believe in inventories so the questionnaire I use does not require scoring of any item. For the past seven years I have been adopting a lifestyle questionnaire originally created by Deanne Jade, Principal of the National Centre for Eating Disorders (UK). The National Centre offers, in my opinion, one of the most comprehensive practitioner training programmes in eating disorders here in the UK and Deanne's questionnaire has proved to be a very useful tool when it comes to sum up all the information gathered during the opening stage. I use the original version with persons who are experiencing eating problems and a simpler version for everybody else – basically the simpler version does not include questions related to eating and dieting.

The lifestyle questionnaire includes the following six sections: general instructions about how to complete it, personal details, medical history, weight history and body image, eating and dieting, and, finally the lifestyle questionnaire itself, which includes eighty personal questions.

Activities Box 19.

Emotional exploration.

Metaphors have been used to help us get the true meaning of our communication across to our interlocutors for thousands of years. The simpler they are, the more effective they seem to be. Confucius, Buddha and Jesus frequently used metaphors to make themselves understood by their contemporaries. Psychologists view them as 'the language of the unconscious' (2), so when, four years ago, I was looking for an interesting and useful way to carry out a brief emotional exploration, I went back to the work of Carl Happich, a German internist, who between 1932 and 1939, developed a technique called 'meadow meditation'. (3)

This consisted of having persons take an imaginary walk through a meadow, up to a mountain, through a forest and into a chapel. Happich viewed the meadow as the youthful mother nature in her serene and beneficent aspect. Climbing the mountain was a symbol of transformation, spiritualisation and humanisation, a movement towards psychic freedom. The forest represented the dark, fearful side of nature, while the chapel the innermost rooms of the person's psyche where the central problems of human life resided.

Happich believed in the archetypal significance of symbols, that is a sort of collective unconscious we all share. In Freudian dream analysis, symbols are produced spontaneously. Through his meadow meditation, Happich would, instead, present his symbols to the person and observe their response.

I did not believe in analysis, nor did I share Happich's unconditional faith in archetypal symbols. At the same time, I wanted to see for myself if I could make any use of Happich's technique and I originated a modified version that I have been employing since.

Starting from the format, the whole exploration takes just two meetings: one for the actual exercise, the other for its discussion. When possible, both meetings are held together. First, I will now illustrate my emotional exploration. Then, I will tell you what meaning I attach to each symbol. Finally, I will openly confess why I have kept on using it and, also why I will, most probably, carry on adopting it for the foreseeable future.

The imaginary walk.

Coming to the exploration, and assuming that I am working with a nice lady, I ask her, first, to describe briefly how does she walk out of her house (i.e. 'walking down the stairs from my third floor flat' or 'taking a lift down from my seventh floor apartment') and if she is used to measuring distances in metres or yards. These little pieces of information will be used at the beginning of her imaginary walk. Then, I ask her if she writes with her right or her left hand – provided I had not already noticed that by myself – and I ask her to position her chair in such a way as to have her non-writing side oriented towards me. I now ask her to assume a comfortable position in her chair.

If I notice that she is not particularly tense, I invite her to close her eyes, close her mouth, and take a few deep breaths. If she looks a bit nervous, I employ a little technique called 'flooding', which consists of having her rational mind carrying out two or three different tasks, at the same time. This way, after a few moments, her rational mind will want to switch off and will allow her to gently close her eyes and be ready to start the exercise. A basic flooding can be to ask her to focus her gaze on a specific point on the wall (1st task), then to invite her to count slowly backwards in her mind from ten to zero (2nd task), and, finally, to have her trying not to blink (3rd task).

When she is there sitting comfortably with her eyes closed, I ask her to carry on with a few deep breaths until she feels more relaxed and, at the same time, I ask her to tell me a simple 'yes', when she does feel more relaxed. When the first 'yes' comes back, I then ask her to visualise herself at **home** and wanting to go for a walk, so I ask her to imagine all the things that she would normally do when she is at home and she feels like going for a walk. I ask her to say 'yes' when she can see herself by the door and ready to go.

On her 'yes', I ask her 'What does your place look like? Does it look messy, tidy or something in between?'

Then, I ask her to see herself walking out of her house – I use now the information provided before to make sure that I don't say anything inconsistent with her real life, like sending her down the stairs when she lives in a ground floor apartment – and, once she can see herself out in the street, I ask her to make her way to the nearest bus stop and to say 'yes' when she is there. Any bus stop would do for the purpose of this exercise. On her 'yes', I ask her to visualise a **bus** coming her way. I tell her not to take any notice where this bus is going, as she wants to explore a part of town she in not familiar with and that is why she will hop on the first bus coming without paying attention to where it is going. So, I ask her to see the bus getting closer, to hop on the bus, take a seat and say 'yes' when all of the above is done.

Now, I ask her to tell me what kind of bus she is sitting in (i.e. old or new, single or double deck), how is the bus maintained (i.e. clean or a bit dirty), what kind of persons are there, where is she sitting, and how does she feel being there. Once I have noted down the answers to the above questions, I then ask her to imagine that after a while she will start realising that the bus has reached a part of town she is not familiar with and I ask her to say 'yes' when she gets this feeling. On her 'yes', I ask her to imagine herself alerting the driver (i.e. pressing the stop button) and getting off the bus. I tell her to say 'yes', when she can see herself back on the pavement again.

On her 'yes', I tell her to walk down some thirty metres until she finds a crossroad. Then, I ask her to look down one of these roads departing from the crossroad and to note in the distance, at the end of the **road**, something that looks like a 'green spot'. I tell her 'it could be anything, because of the distance, that's why I would like you to walk down this road to get to the end of it and tell me what it is, and, as you walk down, could you please tell me what you see on both sides of this road?'

Once I have noted her first impressions of what she can see at both sides of the road, I ask her 'is there anybody there, walking up and down?', 'is anything changing as you walk down on either side?' 'how do you feel walking down this road?' Then, I ask her to visualise that she has reached the end of the road and she is now able to tell what the '**green spot**' is all about. If the green spot is a garden or a park, I ask her to get close. If it is not, then I ask her to walk down turning on one side of her choice (remember that the green spot was at the end of the road, so she cannot walk further up) and to keep walking until she finds a park.

Once she is there close to a **park**, I ask her if the park has got fences around it (and if so, which kind) or is totally open. If she can see fences, I ask her to visualise a gate, and if the gate is closed, I tell her to walk along until she finds an open one. Then, I ask her to enter the park and tell me what she can see, once in there (i.e. what kind of park it is, are there people around, etc.). After I have noted down her first impressions, I ask her to tell me how is the weather and what time she thinks it is now. Then, I ask her to visualise a line of trees and a '**watery spot**' just beyond this line of trees. I ask her to make her way towards these trees, walk past them and tell me what this 'watery spot' is.

I ask her about its shape, size and the colour of the water. I also ask her to tell me something about the state of the water (i.e. if the water is clean, a bit murky or dirty) and if there is anybody around. Then, I ask her to visualise a **bench**. I tell her first to get close to the bench and to describe it to me, and then I ask her to sit on it. Once there, I tell her to relax. I ask her to see herself sitting on that bench, eyes closed, mouth closed, breathing deeply and gently in and out. I tell her to say 'yes' when she feels more relaxed, and on her 'yes' I ask her to see herself standing up and making her way towards a **fountain**, which is not more than thirty-forty metres away.

When she gets close enough to the fountain, I ask her to describe it to me: its shape, material, state, colour and state of water, water flow and, also, if there is anybody else around. Once I have noted all of the above information, I ask her to visualise, 50 or 60 metres away, a **forest**. I ask her to make her way towards it and once there to walk through it and tell me everything she sees once in there. At some point, during her walk through the forest, I ask her 'how do you feel?' and when I have enough information I ask her to see herself almost out of it, and then, eventually, out of it.

As soon as she has walked out of the forest, I ask her to visualise in front of her a hill: she is now at the foot of this hill, standing on a **path** which leads all the way up the hill. I ask her, first, to tell me something about this path, as she walks up the hill, and then to visualise, half-way up the hill, a **house**. Once she sees herself close enough to this house, I ask her to describe it to me. If the place does not look too dangerous or horrific I may also ask her to walk in and tell me how does this place look like from the inside.

Next, I ask her to carry on walking up the hill. I ask her to visualise trees surrounding the top of the hill and a **building** beyond them. Once she is there, **on the top of the hill**, and close to this building, I ask her to describe it to me.

If the building looks safe enough, I ask her to walk in, describe the inside and take a seat. If not, I ask her to visualise a place where she can sit.

Once she is there sitting somewhere, on the top of the hill, I ask her to see herself with her eyes and mouth closed, and I ask her to take a few deep breaths, in and out. When she feels more relaxed, I ask her to tell me how she feels and if there are any particular **thoughts** going through her mind now.

After I have noted this last piece of information, it is time to send her back home. So, I ask her to visualise herself walking down the hill from another side. Then, I ask her to see herself out of this park and waiting near to a little bus stop a few metres away from the park gate. Next, I ask her to imagine a bus coming her way and her hopping on the bus and taking a seat. The bus will first go through an unfamiliar area and then it will take her closer and closer to where she lives, right up to a stop which is very close to her place. Once out on the pavement, I ask her to make her way **back home** and to say 'yes' when she can see herself with her keys in her hand ready to open the door of her flat.

On her 'yes', I ask her to tell me if her place looks exactly how she has left it or if she notices any change (i.e. tidier or messier). Then, I ask her how does it feel to be back home and, finally, I ask her to sit comfortably somewhere, take a few breaths, in and out, and to open her eyes and come back in the consulting room in her own time. I emphasise here that there is no hurry and that she can come back, nice and gently, when she is ready. To help her come back, I adjust my voice now from the soft tone and low pitch used during the imaginary walk to the normal tone and pitch adopted during normal conversation.

The meaning of the symbols.

The second part of the emotional exploration consists of discussing with the person the meaning of the symbols encountered during their walk. Before doing that, I ask them for a brief feedback on the exercise: whether they were comfortable with their eyes closed, were they distracted by any external sound, how was their visualisation, was there anything they saw that they forgot to tell then and can recollect now, etc.

Next I tell them what the exercise is all about, starting from the reason why I ask them to turn their chair. Given that the purpose of this exploration is trying to access their emotional component to acquire some useful information on its condition, our first task is to find a door to access it.

As we have seen above, the practice of bypassing the rational mind by using symbols and metaphors is almost as old as the world itself. Also, medical and psychological practitioners have been using relaxation and hypnotic techniques for almost two centuries now to help persons access and open that door. I do not send people into a state of trance. However, I make sure that they are comfortable and very relaxed before, during and after the whole activity.

Having said that, we can also add that most neuroscientists believe that logical activities are normally (i.e. for persons who are right-handed) associated with the functioning of the left part of the neo-cortex while visual and creative activities are associated with the right one. Whether this is true or not, there is no harm in asking the person to turn and offer to me their left side, if they are right handed – and, naturally, their right one, if they are left-handed. This is because their left hemisphere is directly connected with their right ear, while their right hemisphere is connected with their left ear: as this exercise is about using their visual mode, it would help if my voice would go directly to the right ear. To sum up, according to these neuroscientists, if you would like to engage the person more on a logical level, you are advised to talk directly to the same ear of their handwriting, if you would like to have them accessing their visual and creative level, you are advised to direct your voice to the other ear.

As they offer their feedback, persons commonly note that their visualisation of some of the symbols comes from real objects seen in some real contexts (i.e. the fountain of an Italian town, the bench of a London park, etc.). In these cases I note how, throughout all of their life experience, they have surely seen more than one fountain and more than one bench, and, hence, their emotional self is making a specific choice at this moment in time. In other words, my assumption here is that – though some intrusions from the rational mind are not just possible, but naturally expected – what is talking now is mainly their emotional self.

Let us introduce the specific meaning of each symbol (i.e. home, bus, road, green spot, etc.) However, before that I would like you to note how – though I have carried out this activity more than 150 times over the past four years, I have never come across similar descriptions of symbols.

I say this now, and I re-emphasise the word *never*, because one would normally think that everybody sees the world, more or less like we do: this assumption could not be further from the truth. I was, and still am, fascinated by the apparently endless variety of ways in which each symbol is visualised and described.

I would also like to note how I do not impose my own interpretation of symbols to persons and I always openly discuss their visualisations with them: as a matter of fact, I do not hold a personal interpretation of symbols, for they are not my images we are discussing but theirs! In other words, my task is a simple and limited one: offer them an opportunity to connect with their emotional selves and try to gain an awareness of their condition (i.e. if there are unresolved emotional issues and their impact on the person's life).

First symbol: the person's home.
The first symbol we present is the person's home. We will discuss this symbol at the end because how the person finds their home, on their way back from their imaginary walk, is also our last question and we will comment on the differences between the two described scenarios.

Second symbol: the bus.
The bus is the metaphor for professional life and aspirations. I have had brand new buses and old badly maintained ones. They can also be clean or dirty and the person may feel more or less comfortable being there. It is interesting to note where the person sits and then ask them if there was any particular rational motivation for that, because in the absence of one, which is normally the case, there is something more that we can learn about this person's emotional connection with their professional life and working environment. So, for example, persons with a higher emotional tendency towards control or professional achievement, normally go up to the higher deck and sit in the front row of seats, or sit close to the driver but not on his side, persons more relaxed about their professional life tend to sit towards the centre or the end of the bus, curious persons sit next to the window and those who do not feel particularly secure prefer an aisle seat, travelling companions could be nice people or dodgy-looking types, and the person may feel more or less comfortable being there. Then again, it is always a good idea to check for any rational motivation, first: for example, a tall person may prefer an aisle seat because it provides more leg room. As the person gets more and more into their imaginary walk, however, it is clear how logic and rational motivation give way increasingly to deeper emotional material.

Third symbol: the road.
The road is the metaphor for personal life as it is now. I have had persons telling me that there were high walls on both sides of the road and virtually no pavement – which makes you think of how oppressed they may feel – or there were persons seeing a huge car park but with no cars in it, on the one side, and burnt desolated land, on the other.

Persons may also come up with less bleak representations, such as nice houses or shops and gardens or parks. Likewise they may feel either confused or uncomfortable as they walk down this road or happy and relaxed.

Fourth symbol: the green spot.
This is the metaphor for their emotional connection with Mother Nature – meant both as physical environment (i.e. the natural world: sea, land, sky, etc.) and as social environment (i.e. family, friends, etc.). One might assume that all persons come up with something to do with nature – after all the spot is green – right? Therefore, we would expect trees, gardens, parks and the like. Well, then again, we may be in for many interesting surprises. So, the green spot could also be an advertising board, a big refuse collector, a motorbike, or a statue, just to name a few alternative representations. If the person sees immediately something to do with nature, the emotional connection with Mother Nature is there, at various degrees of quantity and quality, otherwise we can already note how an important connection is not really activated and discuss this with the person.

Fifth symbol: the park.
If the green spot is not a green area big enough to explore, then, as we previously noted, we direct the person to a park, to explore fully their connection with the physical and social component of Mother Nature. For some the park could be an expanse of green grass full of flowers and trees and people engaged in a number of activities (i.e. couples walking hand in hand, mothers playing with children, kids playing with dogs), for others just an open field with nothing to it and nobody around.

Sixth symbol: the time.
The time is the metaphor of the person's emotional age, of how old their emotional self feels. This has nothing to do with their chronological age. Psychologists know that there are different ages to a person and the chronological is not just only one of them, but, also, is the less meaningful when compared to our emotional and rational ages (both at personal and at interpersonal level). So, for example, I have seen fifty-five year old persons making kids' choices and behaving like children, while, to the contrary, I have seen twenty year olds displaying a balanced and wise approach to life and its downturns. I have received a wide range of time references, from very early in the morning (i.e. 5 or 6 am) to very late at night (i.e. 1 or 2 am).

This is very interesting, because it shows how, at this stage of the activity, the emotional voice begins to take over logic. When persons are asked if they were likely to go for a walk in a park at 5 am or at 11 pm, or later, on their own, they all reply that there is no chance they would ever do that! Yet, now that the emotional self has taken over, they feel free to say what is emotionally meaningful, rather than what is logically consistent.

Then again, this exercise is not about looking for something 'wrong' or 'right' with the person: each reference has its meaning and value. So, for example, those who go for a morning time feel that there is a lot of energy at their disposal but, at the same time, this could generate feelings of uneasiness with the current situation. To the contrary, persons who indicate a night time feel that they have been through quite a lot and their emotional batteries are low, but, at the same time, this could favour feelings of satisfaction about their life.

Seventh symbol: the watery spot.
This is the metaphor for how they receive life forces (i.e. love, warmth and affection). I check their watery spot for quantity and quality, to find out if they are sufficiently emotionally connected with their social environment both in term of how many relations they have, but, most importantly, how meaningful they are. The spot (quantity) can be a rain dip, a pond of various dimensions, a stream, a waterfall, even a big lake, and can be man-made or natural. The water (quality) can be clean, clear, naturally murky, a bit dirty or very muddy. As you can see, this metaphor can give a useful indication of the appropriateness of encouraging the person to work either on the quantitative aspect of their relationships, or the qualitative, or both.

Eighth symbol: the bench.
This is the metaphor for how they emotionally relate to material possessions: are they happy to be or to have? If their bench is made of warm material like wood they are not materialistic persons and, at most, they value money or properties not as ends in themselves but for what you can have through them (i.e. buying a house for starting a family, having enough savings to secure your children's education, etc.).

When the bench is entirely made of cold material, like plastic or metal, that means the opposite. When it is made of a combination of both (i.e. wooden slats with metallic arm rests) that signifies a balanced approach between pure idealism and mere materialism.

As I practise in Victoria, central London, at a walking distance from a number of parks (i.e. Hyde Park, St James's Park and Green Park to one end and Battersea Park to the other), persons commonly say to me '…but, Tommaso, I have cut and pasted my bench from this specific park, how can you make this connection with my being more or less materialistic?'

My answer is 'the next time you walk through that park, please take a proper look at the benches there and note if they are all the same, or, if there are different kinds.' I know that each of London's parks have, at least, two different types of benches, some have up to three or four different kinds.

Also, persons' representations may come from a wide variety of sources, from the purely imaginary ones to jigsaw-like representations of a variety of real ones. So the bench may come from a local park as well as from a Spanish sea village and the fountain may come from an Italian town as well as from the London Zoo.

My point is, in the end, our emotional selves choose which ones are going to be visualised.

Ninth symbol: the fountain.
The fountain is the metaphor for how we give life forces. In other words, this symbol mirrors the watery spot. Some may not receive enough, some may not give enough. We may experience considerable emotional pain as a result of a mismatch of these two variables.

So, for example, if you are a 'giver' and receive enough but you feel like you are not giving enough (i.e. the fountain is broken, or very little water comes out of it), this may cause emotional distress. You may be a giver, your fountain is fine (so you are giving enough) but you are not receiving enough (i.e. the watery spot is either too small or the water is muddy), this also may cause emotional distress, because, as a giver, you are required to recharge at some point as keeping on giving for a prolonged period of time will use up a considerable amount of energy.

Similar considerations, but naturally in the opposite direction, may be presented for those who feel more like 'receivers' (i.e. take more pleasure in receiving than in giving). As it appears clear, from the above examples, as always what we are looking for is a balance between the two. The watery spot and the fountain metaphors can help us appreciate how unbalanced we are, when it comes to the specific emotional issues of receiving and giving life forces.

Tenth symbol: the forest.
The forest is the metaphor for the deeper part of our emotional self. It is not the deepest – which is the building at the top of the hill – but we are really beginning to go down now. This could be a pleasant place where the sun is shining through the trees, birds are singing and people are walking their dogs.

However, this could also be one of the places where traumas and major unresolved issues may come up in the shape of ghosts, monsters, scary individuals and darkness. In a couple of cases, the person did not even want to enter the forest and asked me for an alternative way around, which I naturally immediately provided.

Were I practising as an analyst, I would have taken these opportunities to push the person into the forest to confront their demons and I would have worked through the recollection of their traumatic events as they were being re-activated: this is what catharsis is all about.

However, as I am not an analyst and I believe that catharsis is rarely helpful, most times useless and, at times, plainly detrimental to the person's psychological well-being, I prefer to abstain from its application.

The integrated person care way of dealing with distress and traumas is through the resetting of all four components (i.e. physiological, emotional, rational and behavioural): we do not fight the monsters or embrace them as they are.

We, first, get ourselves to a much healthier and safer place, then we get to know them better while always keeping appropriate boundaries. Finally, we make peace with them while, at the same time, gently leading them out of our life.

Eleventh symbol: the path.
The path is the metaphor for the persons' degree of difficulty in dealing with emotional issues. I take care of telling the person at least twice that they are walking up the hill: the path can be a grass-made country footpath or a man-made track, it can be easy to climb, or wet and slippery, it can go upwards gently or it can be represented as the steps of an Aztec temple (a few hundred of them, in a person's case).

Twelfth symbol: the house half-way up the hill.
This house is the metaphor for the person's family. I have had some amazingly pertinent representations here.

I used to receive first with surprise and then with incredulity the visualisations offered, because I could not believe how consistent they were with what I would have found out later, during the discussion with the person.

To offer just a few extreme examples, I have had houses whose number of rooms was exactly the same as that of the family members (nine, in this case!), while the family in question would, in real life, live in a three-bedroom flat, or houses that were exactly like the family's one; houses that consisted just of a few burnt pillars (the lady in question had been continually sexually abused by her uncle when she was a child, had not received any support from her parents, who would not believe her, and, finally, managed to take refuge in a women's centre away from home to stop the abuse once and for all), and houses that looked exactly like the place of work of the person's father.

Most importantly, in over 150 cases, I have never found a person whose later rational recollection of their family was not emotionally consistent with their visualisation. Naturally, the usefulness of this metaphor does not reside in the above degree of consistency – it would be quite a futile symbol and a waste of time and energy, if we were to use it like that – but, rather in the fact that the visualisation of the house allows the person a clear insight into their current feelings towards their families, and, hence the opportunity to put together all the pieces of a jigsaw, which could be very difficult to assemble by using only rational resources.

Thirteenth symbol: the building on the top of the hill.
This is the metaphor for the deepest part of the person's emotional self. Here, we may find our innermost fears or desires. This building can be a nice country house or a scary medieval church, a beautiful villa overlooking a gorgeous panorama or a neglected bungalow. Here, as I ask persons to see themselves sitting somewhere comfortably, I have received some very meaningful and useful answers to my standard question 'are there any thoughts going through your mind now?'

First and last symbol: the person's home.
Differences in how the person finds their home, on the way back from their walk, are a metaphor for the degree of emotional resistance we may encounter when trying to introduce changes in the person's life. So, for example, if the person finds their place exactly as they have left it or even in better condition and they are happy to be back, it means that their emotional self has given the green light to start working on its issues.

If, however, the person find their place in worst condition, that means that it would be appropriate to address the emotional resistance before any other intervention is carried out. I have had homes looking like somebody had been redecorating them or cleaning them up, while the person was away on their imaginative walk, and homes that had been burgled or whose windows had been smashed by vandals.

Why am I carrying out the emotional exploration?

As you have seen, a lot of useful information can be obtained thanks to this activity. Most importantly, is information that we would find very difficult to gain, with such immediacy and accuracy, by means of a purely rational investigation. I am aware that through my adaptation of Carl Happich's meadow meditation some (Freudian and Jungian) analytical concepts have filtered down to this activity. However, I also hope you will have noted how differently I view, relate to and employ these concepts and metaphors. I am also conscious of the fact that, in asking persons to assume a particular position with regards to the direction of my voice, I am utilising knowledge which is commonly applied in Neuro Linguistic Programming (NLP) practice.

I openly confess that I don't have any problem with that! There are 23 steps to the Integrated Person Care process and I welcome the fact that they have not been created entirely as a result of personal inspiration but that they are also based, to different degrees, on pre-existent and consolidated useful knowledge. When a composer creates a new symphony, they do not invent music or its building blocks (i.e. the seven notes). I have never meant to disregard one century of psychological work and research: what I deem useful and helpful has been incorporated into my working model.

The final result begins to appear now before your eyes: only two meetings to delve into the person's emotional depths and to make sense of them. A net saving of a few months (or a few years) of time, energy and financial resources, which can be re-directed towards more beneficial and fulfilling activities.

Activities Box 20.

The Rational Exploration.

The rational exploration is carried out in a couple of meetings and consists of asking the person to create a grid which includes some of their personal constructs. The original version of the repertory grid and personal construct theory were originated by George Kelly in the mid-fifties in the US. I have created my own version of his grid, but before we take a closer look at it, let's first introduce briefly Kelly's ideas.

Kelly believed that we all create personal theories about us and the world and that these theories provides us with predictions about future events guiding our behaviour, just like an internal book of rules. He called these theories 'personal constructs' and maintained that persons are continually engaged in testing and modifying them, just like scientists would do with their working hypotheses.

To elicit personal constructs he created the Repertory Grid Test ('Rep Grid'). This test is a way to help the person discover the fundamental constructs they use for perceiving their life and how they relate to others.

Psychologists generally agree that the Rep Grid stands on its own as a technique, that is, you are not required to share Kelly's views in order to use it. The original version is construed by following the steps below:

(a) write a list of the most important persons in your life (Kelly call these 'elements');
(b) choose three of these elements;
(c) ask yourself 'In what ways are two of these alike and different from the third?' The descriptions given (i.e. my sister and my girlfriend are generous, my uncle is not') offer a construct which is expressed in a bipolar way (i.e. generous – not generous);

(d) this construct is applied to all the remaining elements;

(e) then another set of three elements is selected and the whole process is repeated until a sufficient number of constructs has been identified.

The above process can be reported on a grid whose top horizontal cells are filled in with the chosen elements and the left hand side vertical ones include the personal constructs that are progressively identified. The completed grid will offer an insight into your internal book of rules, which then can be explored in breadth and depth by yourself or by your practitioner.

My adaptation of Kelly's grid is enclosed in Appendix A and it is construed by following the steps below:

a) ask yourself 'What are the first three things (i.e. persons, events, situations) that come to mind when I think about my past?'

b) write down the answers in the first three top element cells of the grid and then repeat the same question for your present and your future, making sure that you are not over-thinking it but that you pick up the first things springing to mind;

c) once all nine elements are entered in their cells, randomly select three of them (I use nine little pieces of folded and numbered paper and ask the person to fish from them) and then ask yourself which two would you put together and why;

d) the 'why' above provides either directly or soon enough (i.e. in some cases you may wish to clarify the point) the personal constructs you are looking for and you enter the constructs in the left hand side cells (the 'similarities' column) and their opposites in the right hand side cells (the 'opposites' column, by 'opposites' I mean what *you* think are the opposites to your personal constructs, not what others may think and these opposites are not associated with the specific elements you have randomly chosen but are simply the result of what springs to mind when you read the words you have entered in the personal constructs cells);

e) once you have completed all of the PCs cells, you are now required to score the grid by allocating a number between 1 and 5 to each cell: when you cross each element with a personal construct, this association may be more or less meaningful, so if an element is very much associated with what is written in the similarities column you score the cell with a 1; when is very much associated with what is written in the opposites column you score the cell with a 5; when an element is fairly associated with the left or the right you go respectively for a 2 or a 4; and, finally, when the crossing of an element and a personal construct does not make sense or you are not sure, you score the cell with a 3.

How do I make sense of the above version of the Rep Grid?

As a practitioner, I don't believe in interpreting somebody else's life and experiences and the way I make use of the above grid is no exception. What counts is the person's view through their own eyes and this is exactly what comes up as a result of completing the grid.

I discuss the grid with the person at two different levels. First, at a 'quantitative level', and, then at a 'qualitative' one.

The quantitative work involves counting how many 'extreme ratings' (i.e. how many 1 and 5 scores) have been expressed. We count them by column (elements) and by row (personal constructs). This simple activity gives us an indication of the elements and constructs with the most 'extreme ratings' and, at the same time, provides us with the total number of 'extreme ratings' as compared to the overall number of cells (i.e. 30 out of 90).

As Gross notes: *Kelly believes that the traditional concept of motivation can be dispensed with. We do not need concepts like drives or needs or psychic energy to explain what makes people 'get up and go' – man is a form of motion and a basic assumption about life is that 'it goes on' 'It isn't that something makes you go on, the going on is the thing itself'. (4)*

The overall number of extreme ratings and the indication of which elements and constructs have more of them, may tell us something about the 'going of the thing itself' both in terms of the person's connection with their own reality and of the sensitivity of some issues as compared to others. My natural assumption would be that if somebody scores very low (i.e. up to 20 out of 90), I would perceive them as disconnected from their reality and I would discuss this with them, without imposing my own view and claiming any expertise on the subject. On the other hand, when somebody scores very high (i.e. 70-75 out of 90), I would be led to think that they feel overwhelmed by their issues and concerns. Then again, I am not interested here in proving or disproving my assumptions, what I observe is the person's response to my observations and how our interaction develops as a result of them.

The qualitative work involves discussing first the personal constructs that have emerged and then asking the person if the opposites chosen represent a 'dictionary opposite' or not. My reason for asking this question is that often the non-dictionary opposites tell a lot about the person's operating mindset. So, for example, a definition opposite of 'happy' would be 'unhappy' or 'sad'. If the person says 'lonely', instead, what do you think this says about them? Once again, I do not jump to conclusions and I would ask them what do they make of their choice of opposites and take it from there.

Activities Box 21.

> Time for your *PAL* …
> *Write down your reflections on the above activity.*
>
> and for your *BIT.*
> *If you are a practitioner, have a go at the rational exploration both as a professional and as a person.*

Discussion.

The opening stage ends with a final discussion where all the activities carried out (i.e. initial consultation, lifestyle questionnaire, emotional and rational exploration) are summarised and integrated to present a whole picture of the person's current situation.

This is when I may ask a few more questions arising from my reading of the lifestyle questionnaire.

Normally one meeting provides sufficient time to do the above and to agree on the way forward.

Activities Box 22.

Time for your *PAL* ...
What do you think of the opening stage, as a whole?

and for your *BIT*
Discuss the opening stage with your travel mate.

Chapter 6

Sensations

> *"Through our senses the world appears.*
> *Through our reactions we create delusions.*
> *Without reactions the world becomes clear."*
>
> *Buddha (1)*

Here we go.

Life is about choices and responsibilities. Reading this book is your choice and it will be entirely up to you whether you will practise what is suggested here. One of the questions I am frequently asked is 'Can I do it?' or 'Will I be able to get through this?' My answer is: $P = M + S$.

P stands for the power to introduce changes in your life. Change is possible provided that you have a combination of M (motivation) and S (skills). How motivated are you? I am talking quality here not quantity. If you are motivated, then I'll show you how to take care of yourself. If you are not quite sure and the motivation seems to be one of the problems, it may be that as you keep on reading this guide the motivation can come through an internal door you never even noticed was there!

Why are we starting from the body? Why don't we go straight into emotional or rational work? *'Mens sana in corpore sano'* (healthy mind within a healthy body), as the Romans used to say. If you normally eat junk food, regularly smoke, heavily consume alcoholic drinks, frequently have tea and coffee and rarely put together seven-eight hours of sleep a night, why are you so surprised if you don't perform as well as you would like to or if you often find yourself in a terrible state of mind? Do I want to take all the fun out of your life? To the contrary, one of the purposes of this guide is to show you how to have plenty of fun and make the most of your life.

Statistics tell us that our life expectancy is improving. Yes, sure. But are our western populations healthier just because we live longer? I remember having read somewhere that when a journalist congratulated the Italian researcher Rita Levi Montalcini when she was awarded the Nobel prize for medicine by saying 'your research will allow us to live longer', she replied 'my dear friend, the point is not to add days to our life, but life to our days'.

This is exactly my point too! I take care of my body not because I want to live forever, but because I would like to be happy and functional for as long as my ticket for this life performance lasts.

How to go about it? This first step will address two topics: glucose level and balanced eating. Then, the second step will show you how to apply what is introduced now and have a great time in the process. Finally, the third step will open the doors to a beautifully integrated and fascinating system: your body!

Activities Box 23.

Time for your *PAL* ...
What do you do to take care of your body?

and for your *BIT.*
Discuss the above with your travel mate.

Sensations

First step
Learning how to take care of your body

Glucose level: haven't you forgotten something?

Why does your glucose level matter? If you don't maintain a stable level of glucose in your bloodstream you may experience any or a combination of the following symptoms: nervousness, shakiness, headaches, feeling miserable for no apparent reason, lack of concentration, and tiredness.

I once saw a person that came to me complaining of tension and nervousness. I could have been a psychoanalyst and asked him to see me three times a week for the next two-three years. I could have been a psychotherapist and offered him a weekly slot for the next twelve months. I could have been an orthodox cognitive behavioural therapist and invite him to participate in a 25-session programme of therapy. For his good luck, I am a psychologist who practises IPC and I saw him for just three meetings. How was this possible? Am I a miracle worker? Of course I am not!

During the initial consultation, I simply asked him 'what do you have for breakfast?' and when he replied that he had been skipping breakfast for the past three years and that the first food entering his body was a Danish pastry at around 10 am, I asked him to have breakfast every day for the whole of the following week and gave him a few hints on how to go about it. When he came for his second meeting a week later, he was already feeling better and I used the second and third meetings to give him more information about the connections between his body and his mind, and that was it! I received an email from him a few weeks later where he confirmed his healthy condition and thanked me for having gone straight to the point.

To make sure that you keep your level of glucose stable, all you are required to do is to have three regular meals a day (i.e. breakfast, lunch and supper), to increase the quality (note, not the quantity) of complex carbohydrates (i.e. good bread, rice, potatoes) and to decrease the quantity of refined carbohydrates (i.e. sugar, cakes, biscuits) and junk food (i.e. crisps, confectionery, etc.). It is as simple as that!

Some say they don't have time for breakfast or lunch. That's a pretty lousy excuse. It takes twenty minutes to have a decent breakfast and you are better off trading twenty minutes in bed for the pleasure of a healthy start to your day: you will sleep better the coming nights if you have a more balanced approach to your daytime activities.

The same applies to lunch. Common excuses are 'I am too busy to have a lunch break' or 'my colleagues don't have one, it may look odd if I start having mine'. I am sure you can think of better things to do with your time and money than seeing a doctor or a therapist and that is where your unhealthy habits have brought you (or will bring you very soon).

You'd better make time for your lunch break, even half an hour is better than nothing and, in time, you will gently and gradually appreciate how important your break is and you will enjoy your full one hour away from work. You will notice that when you take your lunch break nothing terrible will happen: the world will still spin around, the office building will be still standing there, nobody will die as a result of your planned and legitimate short absence and you will actually feel your work performance improve during the second part of the day. After all, they don't pay you to keep your chair warm. They pay you for the quality of your work and your lunch break will improve that quality!

Nobody in the office is having a lunch break? Well, good luck to them! What would you like to do, keep on following them all the way down the cliff, like sheep after a blind shepherd? Do they look like they are all doing fine? Ninety per cent of the persons I see tell me that they put on a brave face at work: they are not doing fine, at all. They just keep going and keep up with sad and unhealthy lifestyle choices. A very successful professional once told me 'I feel like a rat on a treadmill. Always working. Never stopping. Earning a lot. Spending a lot. And at the end of it, what's left? I have been pushing too hard for too long and now here I am, feeling like a wretch.'

Balanced eating: missing information or misinformation?

There are thousands of books out there dispensing information on new and old diets and not surprisingly so. The 'diet industry' is a multi-billion pounds (or dollars) business. Everybody seem to be a winner: book sellers and authors make huge profits, magazines and journalists take their share of the pie and people seem to find the answer to their prayer 'want to look great without much work'.

It stays a great business precisely because, in the long run, none of these diets work and people come back for more: if one of them worked, that would have been it! No more selling and buying, people would know what to do and how to go about it.

In other words, many people make a pretty good living out of exploiting others' laziness and dumbness. Tired of being lazy and playing dumb? Well, here it goes, let's do it!

Obesity is fast becoming a widespread problem in our western societies. However, in the vast majority of cases, it is not due to genetic factors or intervening diseases. So, whether you would like to lose or gain weight it is a simple matter of input (what you allow into your body) and output (what you do with your body). Let's first clarify here some basic points about the input. The next steps will show you how to put them into practice and will also deal with the output part of the equation.

Here is what Dr Robert Lefever, a medical practitioner, says about eating:
"The solution to problems of diet, nutrition and body weight in normal society is primarily to eat a normal, healthy, mixed diet, with three regular meals a day and no snacks in between. Spreading one's food intake to include fats, carbohydrates and proteins is essential. One should have whole grains, nuts, fish and white meat in preference to red, and one should have plenty of fresh fruit and vegetables. That is really all one needs to know. There is no place for supplements and there is absolutely no place for pharmacological substances to stimulate or reduce the appetite. These substances will inevitably be addictive when they are used in an attempt to influence an emotional problem (an eating disorder as such or, alternatively, simple comfort eating, comfort starving or – believe it or not – comfort vomiting or purging) by treating the end results rather than looking at the cause.

Ultimately we should learn to eat according to hunger. Most people do that anyway although they may occasionally have a pork-out or put themselves temporarily on a diet to lose a few pounds for some reason best known to them. For people with eating disorders, however, the idea of eating according to hunger is novel. They would tend to eat or abstain when they are angry, lonely or tired rather than when they are hungry or full. For them the concept that fat comes from food is far from being a statement of the obvious: it is a fundamental challenge to their personal philosophy." (2)

How do you know when you are hungry? Do you eat when your stomach rumbles or when it's time to have a meal? Do you eat when you feel nervous or tired or when you are happy and relaxed?

Being aware of what kind of hunger you regularly experience is already a valuable step in the appropriate direction because it allows you to respond to each stimulus with the proper behaviour. If you are experiencing genuine hunger you'd better eat. If it is an emotional hunger I will show you how to deal with it in the 'emotions' section of this chapter. If you are hungry because you are worried about something, the 'thoughts' section will show you how to address it in a logical way.

If you would like to find out more about what to eat and when, you will find plenty of information in Appendix A (Frequently Asked Questions) and B (General Information). Some people tell me "I know what to do, but I find it difficult to do it." If this is you, you will see how the next steps will offer you advice as to 'how' to take good care of your body.

If you think you are suffering from an eating disorder, please do carry on reading the next step in preparation for the following section ('behaviours'), which will help you stop or, significantly decrease, self-harming behaviours like vomiting, purging or continuous eating. If, however, you are regularly making yourself sick, there is just one thing I want you to know now: the next time you do it, it could be your last!

Yes, you have read correctly. When I ask persons who have been into vomiting for a number of years what damage do they think their behaviour is causing to their health, they mention damage to their teeth and to organs associated with their digestion (i.e. oesophagus, stomach). Nobody ever mentions number one: our heart.

When you make yourself sick, time after time, you are seriously affecting your electrolytes balance (the balance of precious fluid rich in essential minerals which keeps our internal organs functioning like clockwork). Upsetting your electrolytes balance, regularly and severely, as some persons deep into bulimia do, can therefore affect your heart functioning. Simply put, you are playing Russian roulette with it.

Now that you do know the consequences of your behaviour, are you sure this is a game you want to play? Do you really want to keep on risking your life, your very existence on this planet, for the sake of your emotional distress?

The resourcing stage of the Integrated Person Care Programme consists of fifteen steps. Each is designed to help you take care of yourself and of your personal and interpersonal issues. You are warmly invited to embrace the new games you will learn and leave behind the old – and seriously unhealthy – ones.

Activities Box 24.

Time for your *PAL* ...
In taking care of your body, write down a list of ten things that you normally do and ten things that you do not normally do.

and for your *BIT.*
Begin putting the advice above into practice, starting from your daily breakfast and lunch break.

Sensations

Second step
Exploring the connections between body and mind

This step will show you the role played by three brain chemicals (serotonin, endorphin and BDNF) in your overall functioning and how to look after yourself by taking care of your body while having a great time in the process.

Serotonin.

In pop psychology (i.e. articles in magazines, newspapers and self-help books) serotonin is usually depicted as the 'happy hormone'. Well, it isn't really like that! Serotonin is the brain chemical which helps you stabilise your mood and passes on the message "calm down, relax, take it easy". When you visit your GP and get prescribed Prozac, Seroxat or Lustral – that is a Selective Serotonin Reuptake Inhibitor, SSRI – what your little pill does for you is pretty straightforward: it allows you to re-use the serotonin that you are able to produce by inhibiting the functioning of your *cleaner* cells and having the same molecules of serotonin hitting your cell receptors repeatedly.

What many don't know is that you can increase your serotonin level by eating the appropriate food.

As you will see in a moment it is not difficult to do, but, at the same time, it is not difficult to prevent yourself from releasing enough serotonin either.

The little formula you want to keep in mind is $S = C + T + VB6$. To make sure that you are able to release serotonin when required, you want to eat C , that is, complex carbohydrates (i.e. bread, rice, pasta, vegetables, etc). T stands for tryptophan, which is an essential aminoacid found in proteins. Foods rich in tryptophan are: chicken, cheddar cheese, ground beef, tuna, tempeh, cottage cheese, tofu, salmon, scrambled eggs, spaghetti, kidney beans, quinoa, almonds, lentils, milk, soy milk and yogurt. Vitamin B6 is found in almost everything we eat. Foods rich in B6 are: wheat germ, oats, baker's yeast, yeast extract, mackerel, liver, nuts, soya beans, potatoes, bananas, garden peas and green cabbage.

Now, you want to eat all three of the above during the day to do the trick, only two out of three won't do it. As you can see, eating lots of refined carbs and sugary stuff not only messes up your glucose level, but prevents you from releasing serotonin too!

Make sure that you don't overcook or fry your proteins. The more you cook them, the less nutrients you are getting from them. Naturally, I am not asking you to eat raw meat, but steaming, boiling, pressure cooking and grilling (exactly in this order) are much better than frying or microwaving.

When it comes to vitamin B6, many tell me "No problem there, I am having lots of supplements". Well, that could be precisely the problem, instead. You see, eating too much of a particular vitamin may throw your vitamin balance off, resulting, in the long run, in damage to your health. If you are not allergic to certain types of food, my advice is to avoid supplements and get your vitamins directly from their natural sources. If you have a varied and balanced eating style, you will provide your body with all the vitamins it requires.

Endorphins.

Now, these are what we might call 'the happy hormones'. Research has shown that endorphins make us feel good about ourselves and a number of studies have associated endorphins with raised confidence and self-esteem. So how do we get them flowing through our system? There are, at least, six ways to help our bodies release endorphins and, not surprisingly, they are all connected to our senses (the psychological word for 'sense' is 'modality'). Let's introduce them, one by one.

1. Food.
Yes! Here we go again. Your sense of taste can induce powerful pleasurable responses. A recent survey showed that women in the UK preferred chocolate to sex: sad but true! So, how to go about it? The idea here is to make your eating pleasurable without having necessarily to favour sweet or very savoury foods. In other words, you are encouraged to begin appreciating food for its natural taste, rather than over-spicing it. Make every eating moment a pleasurable one starting from your sight (i.e. put a nice table cloth down, choose cheerfully coloured plates). Then, have some flowers on your table and put your favourite music on.

Most importantly, eat slowly. You want to feel the taste of what you are eating. Fast eaters are more likely to become binge eaters, feel bloated or have digestive problems. Apply the ancient Buddhist rule "Eat as you were drinking and drink as you were eating". That is, properly chew your food and swallow it when it's almost liquid and drink in sips.

I used to be a very fast eater myself and I have steadily and gradually changed this unhealthy habit by initially leaving my fork or spoon on the table each time I had used it to place food in my mouth. I would pick it up again only when I had properly masticated and swallowed what I had in my mouth first. It felt a bit weird, at the beginning, but it worked! Now, I can hold cutlery in my hand *and* eat slowly, at the same time.

2. Exercise.

Exercising is a well-known way to induce the release of endorphins so much so that some can actually overdo it, like people experiencing anorexia who get the 'runners high'. The healthy approach to exercising is to make sure it is easy and natural. Do it when, how and where you feel like doing it and do not push yourself too hard. You are not competing for the next Olympic games and you are not a professional athlete. I have actually met persons that were even stricter in their exercise routine than professional athletes, by exercising too intensively and by not allowing their bodies enough weekly breaks. So, how much is enough?

You want to use your body **every day** for twenty minutes (two ten minute walks would do). Regularity is the key. There is not much point in killing yourself in the gym for two hours and then spending the rest of the week on your sofa in front of the TV. Besides, exercising occasionally can actually seriously damage your health. Couch potatoes that once a week go crazy on a football pitch or a tennis court play Russian roulette with their hearts. Now you know. Don't risk a heart attack. If you feel like having fun with your friends for the occasional game, make sure your move your body every day to get ready for it.

Do I hear your usual excuse again? "I would love to but I have no time". Set your alarm clock ten minutes earlier and walk around your house or walk around your office block, before and after work.

Do not do the 'stressful walk', that is, going from A to B at your highest speed, wearing high heels shoes and thinking of your bills, your mortgage, your car, your job and your love life, at the same time.

Do the 'nice and easy walk', that is, going from A to B by starting slowly and then gently increasing your pace and then gradually decreasing it, wearing comfortable shoes (you can always get changed once in the office, and yes, I share responsibility for a good deal of those ladies around wearing trainers on their way to work and back home) and think of nothing, just enjoy feeling your body move and if you feel like you require a bit of practice to be able to do that, well, just think of your next holiday or that at the next sharp corner you may bump into your favourite film star.

The regular practice of Peaceflow can also provide a pleasurable alternative to more traditional forms of exercise.

3. Music.
Listening to your favourite kind of music does help you release endorphins too, so go for it. Get yourself a portable CD or cassette player and enjoy it!

4. Laughter.
There may be days when something really funny happens or one of your colleagues keeps on cracking one great joke after another. There may be days when not even a little smile crosses your face. Why is that? Laughter is healthy, so make sure that you create a 'humour corner' at home and at work. Your humour corner at home will have a sample of the things that make you laugh (i.e. books of quotes, jokes, prose, cartoons, DVDs or videos). Make sure that when you are back from work that is the first place you visit. Pick something and have a laugh. This will also help you close mentally your working day and start your personal time.

5. Relaxation, meditation or prayer.
I have placed them together because, depending on your religious beliefs and lifestyle you are obviously free to decide which ones are for you. I will teach you some relaxation techniques, as part of the emotional management programme. If you are already into meditation or prayer, now you have one more reason to practise it.

6. Sex.
Well, 'dulcis in fundo' (the sweet part in the end), we make love. Next time your partner plays difficult, you just tell them that it's for your psychological health (you may wish to bookmark this page, just in case).

Brain-derived neurotrophic factor (BDNF).

BDNF is a brain chemical that, among other things, helps brain cells in the hippocampus regrow, thus counterbalancing the damage done by the stress hormone cortisol. To raise your BDNF levels you can:

1. Exercise.
(see point above and Peaceflow)

2. Eat omega-3 oils.
Oily fish (salmon, herring, mackerel, sardines), walnuts, olive oil.

3. Have acupuncture.

Activities Box 25.

Time for your *PAL* ...
Write down a list of the things that you already do to take care of your glucose, serotonin, endorphin and BDNF levels.

and for your *BIT.*
Begin putting the advice above into practice, by making a plan of how you would like to introduce, nicely and gradually, those changes in your lifestyle which will allow you to release enough serotonin, endorphins and BDNF to keep you out of trouble.

Chapter 7

Behaviours

"It is not our preferences that cause problems,
but our attachment to them."

Buddha (1)

Third step
Prevention is better than cure

This step will first explain what 'behavioural self-help' is about and why it works. You will then be introduced to three practical applications: the Magic Box, the Magic Purse and the Holy Place.

Please bear in mind that the following behavioural self-help techniques serve the purpose of providing an immediate support for when you are frequently experiencing the reoccurrence of unhealthy or self-harming behaviours (i.e. vomiting, self-cutting or withdrawing from social encounters). You will be in a position to comprehensively address your issues – not only the behaviours – only once you will have gone through the learning process associated with the whole of the phemiological person care programme.

The following letter was emailed to me by a girl in her early 20s, who wants to get over her bulimia. I think it offers you a clear idea of what can go on in our mind, at times, and of why behavioural self-help interventions may be appropriate at the very beginning of the person care process.

"I have thought about your question 'What does bingeing do for me?' and came up with the following:
It gives me something to do. This sounds terrible as it is such a waste of my health for such a silly reason, but it is part of the answer. If I am worried about something (usually work or my knee) and want to avoid these feelings then this is the way I usually occupy myself and blot out the thoughts.

The same goes for being stressed/angry/upset.

It helps to keep me in the same place. Part of me is scared of progressing at work or meeting new people by going out, or doing any other positive thing, and so I make myself sick as it keeps my self esteem in a low place. I can hide behind my eating disorder and not face up to the challenges of the real world.

As I have done it for many years now, it gives me security. I have binged many times without wanting to because I have been too scared to stay in the 'real world' and see what happens.

It stops me from missing dancing. I am scared that if I go for long enough without being sick, I will become more in tune with my body and its need to dance. And then I will have to face up to the fact that my dream of a dancing career is never going to happen because my knee is such a mess. The more I am sick, the more numb I feel and the easier it is to cope with the fact that I can't dance."

Help yourself!

I have seen persons who were fully aware of their problems and knew fully well what to do. However, they asked for help in actually applying their knowledge to their everyday life. So, for example, I have worked with nutritionists and dieticians who knew what to eat and were dispensing sound advice every day to their clients, but then Dr Jekill turned into Mr Hyde and they would engage in bulimic or obsessive-compulsive behaviours. The same applies to other health professionals whom I have seen, who got themselves into drinking, drug abuse, smoking and gambling.

How is it that, even when we know that what we are doing is terribly wrong, we feel like we 'cannot' stop the urge to self-harm?

There are two mindsets within each of us and these two 'persons' represent two very different sets of values: the inner adult and the inner child. Those of you familiar with Eric Berne's transactional analysis are advised that these two 'persons' are very different from Berne's ego states (i.e. the internal metaphors of parent, adult and child).

The IPC view is that the inner adult is wise and takes time to consider things and situations. It is logical and able to deal with problems in an effective and rational way. Its downside is that, if left on its own, it can lead us into over-thinking and overworking. The inner child, to the contrary, is the emotional and impulsive part of us. It is creative and has plenty of energy. However, it can get restless, is not interested in the future and by demanding immediate satisfaction NOW can become edgy and scream for attention.

When we try to be too good (i.e. perfectly sticking to a diet, impeccably going about our house work, precisely planning our day and week, etc.) the inner adult places too much pressure on the child, who sooner or later will either implode or explode. Normally, nicer persons tend to implode, turning all this unhealthy energy onto themselves because they are sensitive and considerate individuals who will never hurt someone else, so they end up harming themselves (i.e. bingeing and vomiting, starving, self-cutting, etc). Others explode, instead, and turn this energy against somebody else (i.e. hitting, swearing, threatening, plotting, etc.). The more pressure the adult puts on the child, the more powerful – and seemingly incontrollable and unstoppable – its reaction will be. That's why we feel like we 'cannot' stop the self-defeating behaviours, once we get started.

So, this is how it comes. Now, let's see how it goes.

If a real child was sitting in a room playing with one of the many toys piled up beside her and you were to enter and place close to her a new toy, what do you think her reaction would be? I tell you that a real child would go and play with the new toy, at least for a while, out of curiosity. Does your inner child want to play an unhealthy game, yet again? Is she screaming for attention? Fine. Let's introduce new games for her to play. Let's hear what she wants to say. Let's channel this vast amount of energy into new equally exciting but less harmful activities.

The Magic Box.

The Magic Box will help you choose something else to do, rather than going straight for the self-harming behaviour. This self-help activity is designed for use at home. Before you use your Magic Box you want to create it. First, jot down a list of activities whose two main characteristics are:

> 1. they will keep you engaged for 5 to 15 minutes;
>
> 2. they are exciting, pleasurable or fun.

Thinking of your senses may help you with your list. For example, hearing can attract items like listening to your favourite song or singer, touch can attract items like rubbing your hands with a particular piece of cloth or hand-cream.

Once the list is made, write the items, one by one, on separate little pieces of paper and fold them. Now buy or make a nice box (the nicer the better), one with a proper lid and place your little pieces of paper in the box.

The next time you feel like your inner child is taking over, all you want to do is say to yourself "Ok. I am going to go for a big binge (or whatever your usual self-harming behaviour) in a moment, not just now" and, as you are saying this, you reach for the Magic Box, lift the lid, fish an item and carry out the activity indicated on the little piece of paper. In 75-80% of cases, fishing once is enough for not wanting to go back to the original self-harming behaviour. In the remaining cases, fishing twice does the trick. I have been passing on this technique for the past four years and it has never happened so far that somebody has had to fish three times or that after the second fishing they went back and carried out the unhealthy behaviour.

Why does this simple technique work? We do know that self-harming urges are very powerful. At the same time, we also know that they are extremely transient: that is, once you manage to keep your mind off them for a while by introducing a *response delay,* they pass and go, provided that you don't stage a fight *against* them. If you fight, the inner child will win nine times out of ten and not because you are weak or hopeless or stupid, but because your inner child is in the here-and-now and the wise inner adult is in the future.

Another reason why the inner child will not respond to the rational adult is because when your urge comes about you get to a different place and the language spoken by your inner adult will be incomprehensible to the child in you. In these moments it is extremely difficult to think straight. I know this and that's why I am not asking you to think straight. What I would like you to do is to first acknowledge what is going on and calm down the child by saying "Ok. I am listening to you. I am going to do as you wish, in a moment" and then give the child a new game to play.

In other words, you are trading an immediate behavioural response (i.e. going to the fridge) for another immediate behavioural response (i.e. going to the Magic Box). Even if you find it difficult to talk to the child and calm her down or you forget and go straightaway to the Magic Box, the alternative will still work because it will engage your inner child who will be very happy to fish and play new games.

The Magic Purse.

The Magic Purse is the outdoor version of the Magic Box. You may find it very useful when you are at work. You create the Magic Purse and use it exactly as you do with the Magic Box by unzipping the purse as you would lift the box's lid. The only difference is that the list of activities here are required to be compatible with your work environment. As self-harming behaviours at work tend to come about during the lunch break, you won't find it difficult to create a list of alternative activities to carry out. Frequently items re-occurring on people's lists are: listening to their favourite music on portable CD players, exploring shop windows (and occasionally buying something, as a special treat), planning weekends or holidays. As you progress through the next steps you may add some of the new self-help techniques you will learn to your Magic Box or your Magic Purse.

The Holy Place.

Whether you are at home or at work, you can help yourself by introducing another *response delay* by choosing a place which, from that moment, becomes your Holy Place: that is, a place where, no matter what, you are going to go and spend two to three minutes each time your urge comes about. Your Holy Place is an environment where you feel safe, comfortable and relaxed. It can be a chair, a sofa, a bed, a corridor, a flight of stairs or a room. Some of the persons I have worked with have found it useful to go immediately to their chosen place (as an immediate behavioural response) when they felt the unhealthy urge coming, before doing anything else, because from that place it was then much easier to move on to the next helpful behaviour.

Activities Box 26.

Time for your *PAL* …
Write down a list of the items to place in your Magic Box and Magic Purse. Think about what environment could become your Holy Place.

and for your *BIT.*
Practise the response delay techniques above.

Behaviours

Fourth step
Feeling Peckish?

When you are going through a difficult time, you may wish to remind yourself of the word 'Peckish' which is an acronym for:

Prevention
Exercise
Change
Keep in mind your new you
Ignore specific goals
Solving skills
Have fun

The word **Prevention** is there to remind you that there is so much you can do to avoid getting yourself into difficult situations, which are likely to trigger unwanted behaviours. So, for example, if you are a single guy and your issue is night bingeing and cravings for sugary stuff, why do you buy chocolate biscuits and keep them in your cupboard? I can hear you saying "I have bought them for my friends". Yes, right.

You see, the point is, there are no such things as little elves visiting your home at night and filling your cupboards and fridge with food. *You* have bought what is there in your house. So the next time you walk in a supermarket, make sure that you write *beforehand* a list of what you would like to buy, otherwise you will hear the little voices of many unhealthy foods calling your name (oh, yes, you know they call you by your first name). The reality is that each time you walk in a supermarket you are totally unaware of half of the things you end up buying and regularly forget half of the things that you wanted to buy before getting there.

How come? Are you so dumb? Of course, you are not! Truth is there's a lot of people working behind the scenes to make sure that when we enter a supermarket we buy a lot, and a lot of what *they* would like us to buy. These people know how to run their business.

The whole process that sees a product from its creation to its place on a shelf, from advertising to packaging, from deciding its name and size to its retail price, involve lots of fine minds, including psychologists too! That's why if you want to defend yourself from their tricks and traps, write your list at home and then, once in there, just follow your list and you will be fine.

Another practical example of *prevention is better than cure* is that of what to do during your daily breaks when you are a student. Many students I have worked with go directly to the kitchen and grab something to eat and this frequently triggers binges and subsequent vomiting or purging episodes. They are all bright individuals but when these moments come they all turn into Mr Hydes. In such cases it helps to write down, beforehand, a list of pleasurable and fun activities to carry out during breaks from study or work. So, when the time for a break comes, all you do is to have a look at the list and pick what you fancy at that time, rather than wandering like zombies towards the kitchen.

We have already talked about **Exercise**, so this is just a reminder to go for it, nicely and gently, but on a daily basis.

Change is there to remind you that if you are here, reading this book, it is because you are not entirely satisfied with your life, or, if you are a psychological practitioner, because you would like to learn something new. I normally find it useful, at this point, to present the Karpman's drama triangle. I do this to make you aware of the vicious spiral you may be stuck in and, hence, of the basic fact that change is desirable.

Draw a triangle and write next to the top angle the word 'rescuer', then write next to the lower right angle the word 'persecutor', and, finally, write next to the lower left angle the word 'victim'.

Some of us can get stuck in the following spiral: we start by taking care of people's responsibilities for them (rescuer) and then get angry with them for what we have done (persecutor), and, subsequently, feel used and sorry for ourselves (victim) and to feel better we start taking care of others responsibilities again (back to rescuer). Naturally, we may start from any of the three above 'roles' and once in the spiral we find it difficult to get out. In my experience, many start from feeling victims and then when they have had enough turn into persecutors, but they soon feel bad about it and start playing the rescuers until they become disillusioned and fall into a victim state again.

Whichever way you look at it, one thing is for sure: neither of these three roles is healthy. This person care programme will show you how to break the vicious spiral and look after yourself *and* others in an appropriate way.

Keep in mind your new you, means that if you would like to become a more balanced and happy person it would help if you were able to visualise yourself as the person you would like to be some time in the near future. In order to do that, you may practise a simple and effective technique, which I have called the **K-technique**. I would advise you to go through the following steps one at a time (i.e. one step a day).

First, sit comfortably, close your eyes and imagine yourself in the near future. You look happy and you are in a nice place, either on your own or with somebody. You are the person you would like to become. It doesn't matter if the picture is in black and white or in colour, or if it looks like a photo or it feels like a 3D image. What counts is that the image is clear and is right there at the centre of your inner screen. Then, open up your eyes and write down an accurate description of your image (which from now on we will call, your 'K-image'). Now, read through your written account of the K-image, then close your eyes again and visualise it. At this point you are ready for the final step, which is, you are now able to visualise your K-image with your eyes open. You may try, for example, to 'place it' on your desk or anywhere you like.

How do you use your K-image, once you have created it and practised its visualisation? What is its practical purpose? To illustrate how the K-image can help in real life situations I offer you the typical scenario of a professional woman who spends a good deal of her time at work between the meeting room (i.e. briefings, seminars, negotiations, etc.) and the staff room. Here in England meeting rooms are designed to abide by the following order of priority:

1. Tea and biscuits (necessary)
2. Furniture (basic to minimal)
3. People (optional to irrelevant)

So there you are in the middle of a boring presentation and the tray full of cheap biscuits is looking at you…it's having a laugh…it's calling your name…gosh, what are you going to do? Are you going to think that summer is coming and your skirt is getting despondently tighter? Are you going to remind yourself that if you pick just one biscuit, then a few others will follow?

For a while you will play the yes or no game. Shall I have one or shall I pass? Suddenly, almost by magic, the first biscuit materialises in your mouth, you are virtually unaware of how it got there. Then, a few others follow, and some more find their way from the tray to their new home. Next, you feel disgusted with yourself. How can you be so weak? And the self-blaming game begins.

You see, in the real life example above the unhealthy choice (biscuits, cigarettes, drinks, etc.) does not meet a proper challenge: it's a very strong *you* in the present (I am bored, stressed, tired, nervous) against a weak *you* in the future (if I eat this rubbish I will keep putting on weight, smoking and drinking will damage my health). Moreover, it is the inner child against the inner adult. When you feel bored, stressed, tired or nervous, the inner adult is most likely to give way to the inner child. You want satisfaction NOW and go for the unhealthy choice.

The K-technique introduces what you are looking for: a real challenge to the naughty child, a proper contestant. When you visualise the K-image next to the tray of biscuits, you can see you smiling and happy on one side and the tray of cheap biscuits on the other. That will remind you that this is your life and you do have a choice, whether to get one step closer to the new you, the happy person you would like to become (the slimmer, non-smoking you), or to feed the unhappy person you are now and turn to the cheap biscuits (cigarettes or drinks), thus going back to the downward vicious spiral of self-blame, guilt, low self-esteem and more unhealthy behaviours.

Some blow up the K-image to a bigger size than the tempting unhealthy choice, to make it more powerful. Others may even talk and ask their K-image questions. Naturally the conversation goes on in their minds if others are around. If you are motivated or patient enough to create your K-image and practise its visualisation, you will reap your reward.

Why does the K-technique work? It works because when you visualise and connect with your K-image, you are accessing your inner wisdom, that is, someone or something (depending on the points of view) that will always guide you towards healthy, useful and helpful places. I personally, visualise my K-image every morning on my kitchen table, when I am having breakfast. It helps me stay focussed on my next goal and when I get there I create a new image. Visualising my K-image regularly also helps, because if and when I feel like using it, I am able to place it where I would like it to be quite easily.

Ignore specific goals simply means: it is ok to have plans, but if they are too detailed, you may end up setting the scene for a big disappointment if you fall short, even slightly, of your target.

Solving skills is there to remind you that there is so much you *can* do to get out of difficult situations, once you find yourself in one of them. It's never too late to start taking care of yourself. This guide will provide you with plenty of tools to do that.

Have fun simply means that you can be very good at what you do, personally and professionally, while, at the same time, embracing a light-hearted approach to your everyday chores and affairs. The heaviness and seriousness so often associated with some of the roles we play in life, does nothing to improve the quantity or the quality of our performances, but it does take a toll on our health.

Activities Box 27.

Time for your *PAL* …
Reflect on the PECKISH system above: how many of the ideas introduced here are you already practising?

and for your *BIT.*
Create your K-image and practise the K-technique.

Behaviours

Fifth step
Relapse management

Relapse management is normally the last module of any programme of psychological intervention. But this is IPC, and you might have already gathered by now that we do things in a slightly different way from our orthodox colleagues. Fear not, the fourteenth and fifteenth steps will provide some final 'relapse management' tips. However, there is a point I would like to make now, while we are still at the beginning of our journey.

Do not assume that successful recovery from your problem means that you will *never* go back, even for one single episode, to the behaviour, or feeling, or concern that brought you here in the first place. This will be like digging a hole in which sooner or later you will fall down and hurt yourself. I am not denying that some people may never go back. I am saying that we are humans, not computers that once programmed or re-programmed carry on like that forever. So the point is not whether we may relapse occasionally into an unhealthy behaviour. The point is what we do if and when we relapse.

If you were used to smoking 40 cigarettes a day and then you gradually decrease to 30, 20, 10 a day until you quit altogether, how do you deal with one cigarette smoked three months later? If you see it as a failure, as a sign of weakness, you are in for big trouble. Because if you start the self-blaming game again, you get back into the downward vicious spiral, where the next steps are 'I am worthless', 'I am a lost cause', 'What's the point?' and in no time you will be back to 40 cigarettes a day again.

If, however, you see it as a sign that you are a human being, and as such you are fallible and not perfect, you will be more likely to consider how you haven't smoked one cigarette for three months and that you are capable of waiting, at least, another three months for the next one, if the occasion will arise.

In the end, what counts is that you keep the motivation to look after yourself. You want to congratulate yourself on what you have managed to achieve and keep on looking forward.

Then again, I am not saying that we are all bound to go back, sooner or later, though episodically, to our issues. Some don't and that's great! Nevertheless, we all better keep in mind that life is a process, where we experience given events and situations and learn from them.

So, let's stay focussed on the process and on our learning abilities, rather than on single episodes.

Activities Box 28.

Time for your *PAL* ...
Reflect on the point introduce above: how would you know when you have become the person you would like to become? How would you define the goal of this person care programme?

and for your *BIT.*
Discuss the above with your travel mate.

Chapter 8

Emotions

"Learn to respond, not react."

Buddha (1)

Sixth step
Recognising your emotional states

Getting ready.

The first question I would like you to ask yourself is 'Where do you think emotions come from?'

You may say 'from my mind' or 'from the external environment'. Naturally, we do know that, in the end, all incoming stimuli and information are processed by our brain. However, it may be helpful to note here that at times we are aware of how some feelings come from an internal place (i.e. you wake up in the morning feeling happy or sad) while other times they seem to come from external sources (i.e. the computer that crashes and drives us mad, the colleague making a stupid remark that triggers an angry response).

Identifying the perceived source of a given emotion can be very useful, because it can help us deal with it appropriately. Generally speaking, most of us don't have a clue about how to deal with emotions. This is not because we are weak, stupid or faulty. This is simply because we are taught Geography, History and Maths and we are not taught how to take care of some of our basic life processes. We learn about places 10,000 miles away from home and about events that happened 2,000 years ago and we learn nothing about ourselves. I love Geography and History, so don't get me wrong. However, I would have loved the opportunity to have had somebody coming to my class at least once a month to teach me how to take care of my body, how to deal with my emotions and how to address my rational concerns.

So, let's start by making this guide available in school libraries, and see if we can teach our students how to become more balanced and happier people.

If you are going somewhere, it helps to know where you are going to. You are more likely to get there, I suppose. So, what is the goal of learning emotional management? Well, for a start, this is not about brainwashing or re-programming. Emotional management is about learning how to deal with emotions in such a way as to not upset ourselves and others more than it would be appropriate – depending on the specific life event. We do not fight negative emotions, we let them come in, we observe them, and we show them the way out: this way we don't offer them a permanent place to stay within ourselves. They will stay only for the time necessary for our system to process them.

Our goal is graphically illustrated in figure 1 below.

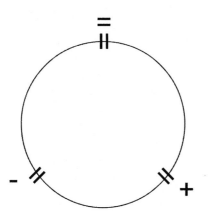

Figure 1. The Emotional Management Process

As you can see, our goal is to get you, first, from a mental place where you are experiencing negative feelings (-) to a place where you feel much more relaxed and calm (=). Then, I will show you how to move from the peaceful place to a happier one (+). This is, by no means, the end of the story. This is just how we are going to progress through the emotional level. There is a healthier, more useful and helpful territory for you to be in and the thoughts section of our person care programme will show you how to get from your happy emotional place to this wonderful new land.

Some people ask me 'why can't we get directly from the negative place to the positive one?' as it does look like you are doubling the journey when you move first to the peaceful place.

Well, in real life sometimes shortcuts are not always as convenient as they may appear to be at first sight. As humans, we greatly benefit from getting first to a calmer place as a healthy way of processing negative feelings. Being at peace, is a great place for you to be: happiness is like a flash of lightning, it comes, gets you high and then returns to the universe. Peace, instead, is a place which you can inhabit.

Also, when you are feeling really low, what do you think your response will be if somebody were to remind you of times when you were very happy? You are most likely to feel even more the gap between where you are now and where you have been (or could be now or in the future, if you weren't feeling that miserable) and this will hurt even more. The recommendation of going about your person care 'nicely and gently' does not apply only to your daily exercise routine: it is valuable advice worth applying to how we deal with our emotions too.

How have you been dealing with your emotions so far.

There are three different ways in which we can respond to emotional material. We can call these ways 'modalities' to help remind ourselves that we do have a choice as to which one we would like to apply to our everyday life circumstances. As you will see in a moment, most of you will deal with emotions by using the first two modalities. I will then introduce you to a third modality and show you its benefits when compared to the others.

First Modality: Action-Reaction Mode.

Sometime we respond to emotional material by reacting to it. We can do so in three different ways: we may lash out, take in or displace.

Lashing out.

When we lash out at somebody who has been abusive or whom we view as the cause of our current emotional distress, we are simply trying to throw the negative emotional energy back to where it comes from.

So, although we may hit back for many different reasons, when we lash out our response is direct and explicit: direct, because there is no time-gap between the emotions impacting on us (action) and our reaction; explicit, because we openly and clearly display our emotional state.

Pop psychology publications may suggest lashing out in a controlled way (i.e. punching a pillow) as a way of releasing tension or anger. Such recommendations are pure nonsense! When we punch a pillow we are teaching ourselves that it is ok to punch and, in so doing, we are consolidating the use of a violent and unhealthy behaviour. Today we punch a pillow. Tomorrow we may punch a person.

There is no place in civilised societies for 'justified violence'. This is what I once read on the subject:

"Intentions, of course, are always good. The worse the fight, the higher its justification. 'Justified' violence is the worst. Unjustified violence bursts out of a bad character or bad feelings, but it doesn't go very far. But when people feel justified in the use of violence, it becomes systematic and leads to all the horrors of history." (2)

"The harmonious development of a child's personality, which insures that he/she embraces the values of peace, tolerance and co-existence, cannot be achieved by using violent means which contradict these goals (such as the parental use of corporal punishment)". (3)

Taking in.

We may respond to emotional material in a direct and implicit way. We minimise the importance of what is happening to us or try to ignore it altogether. We don't show our feelings and, most of the times, don't even share our emotional states with somebody close to us. We 'bottle things up' as they say in British English.

The emotional material does not vanish just because we have decided to ignore it. So, where does it go? We are simply sweeping it under the carpet, or to use another metaphor, we are letting it sink deep down in our emotional container, day after day, week after week, month after month. Then one day we wake up, we feel miserable and depressed. We feel that 'we have had enough' and we don't know what's going on. We have allowed these small time-bombs to sink in and now they are going off. We have lost track of hundreds of 'non important' feelings we failed to acknowledge at the appropriate time and now they have become a big scary ghost who has come back to haunt us.

Displacing.

We may also redirect (displace) the emotional material that life throws at us onto somebody or something else rather than addressing it directly. This happens when, for example, negative emotions originate in the work environment and we displace them onto our partner at home or vice versa, or when we displace our boredom or sadness by eating or drinking compulsively or by starving ourselves.

When we displace, on the one hand, we don't deal with the original negative emotion and, hence, we maintain the source of personal distress, while, on the other, we create new negative emotions by placing unnecessary pressure on ourselves or others.

Second Modality: Action-Proaction Mode.

'Proactive' is an American word initially used in business, which has then leaked into common spoken English. While trying to be one step ahead of the competition may serve a commercial purpose in the workplace, it does not make much sense when it comes to dealing with our emotions. We can be proactive in two ways: by keeping on interrupting our interlocutor, or by daydreaming.

Interrupting.

Every time two humans interact there are at least three channels exchanging information, which gets activated. We sense the other's presence with our body, we get in touch with their feelings, we rationally engage with them. When we keep on interrupting our interlocutor our body is still there, but we respond emotionally and rationally *before* the other has had the chance to complete what they are saying (action) and, hence, our response starts *before* we can receive a full account of what the other really means to say or to do.

Now, how can we appropriately deal with emotional material if we are not fully aware of what is happening to us? When we interrupt our interlocutor we are only making ourselves emotionally vulnerable.

The 'other' may have a communication style whereby they normally start with the good news (i.e. paying you a compliment, or saying something positive about your contribution to a project) and then they bring in the bad news (i.e. saying what they don't like about you, or criticising some of your professional choices).

If you interrupt and start your emotional response after the good news you are exposing yourself to the full impact of the bad news. Others have a communication style whereby they usually start with the bad news and then they introduce the good news. If you interrupt and start your emotional response after the initial criticism you will find it very difficult to accept the good news (if you ever get to hear it, that is!).

Daydreaming.

We all switch off from reality and switch on daydreaming mode for a while during the day. There is nothing unhealthy about it. However, some people spend long periods of time in 'daydreaming mode' and some use it as a regular way of dealing with emotions. When the latter applies we allow our response to start – that is, switching off and landing in a parallel dimension – *before* we can be fully aware of what is happening around us. The real life event is still going on and we decide to leave and go somewhere else.

The more time we spend in our fantasy land and the more energy we put into making it a wonderful place to be, the less time and energy we have to make our real life a more exciting, stimulating and rewarding place to be. Over time our fantasy land becomes a black hole which sucks in the best of us and leaves behind an everyday life ever more ordinary, dull and miserable.

As I have just said, a little bit of daydreaming can be useful and I will show you in due course how to make the most of it when you feel like switching off. However, some people escape life and hide in their parallel dimensions as a way of dealing with negative feelings and this is not healthy, nor helpful.

How to deal with your feelings in a healthy, useful and helpful way.

When we experience negative feelings the 'smoke detectors' in our emotional brain (the amygdalas) go off. Now, if we were to deal with a real smoke detector going off at home because we left a pan of boiling water in the kitchen, we would follow the steps below:

- ✓ switch off the hob
- ✓ throw away the water
- ✓ open the window to let the smoke out
- ✓ manually disconnect the smoke detector
- ✓ make sure that there's no smoke left in the room
- ✓ reset the central fire alarm system
- ✓ manually re-connect the smoke detector

When we are dealing with emotional distress, instead, what do we do? As we have just seen, we may:

- ➢ scream at somebody or hit something as we convulsively deal with the pan (lashing out)
- ➢ pretend nothing is happening (taking in)
- ➢ go down to the pub for a few drinks (displacing)
- ➢ have a chat with a justifiably worried neighbour (interrupting)
- ➢ think about our next holiday (daydreaming).

We have seen so far how *not to* respond to negative emotions. The following section and the next three steps will show you how to deal with them.

Third Modality: Action-Preaction Mode.

First of all, what does 'preaction' mean? The 'pre' stands for 'preventative' and for 'preliminary'.

Preventative, because if you decide to follow my advice you will not get into trouble by lashing out, taking in, displacing, interrupting or daydreaming. There is only one of you and if you direct yourself in one direction, you will not be able to get somewhere else, at the same time. Imagine you are in a big room and there are six doors in front of you.

If you open and go through one of them, you won't be able to enter any of the remaining five doors simultaneously. Many develop physically before they are ready mentally and in such cases it is very important to wait and give ourselves the opportunity to choose the proper *way in* our emotional self.

Preliminary, because when you go through the appropriate door, you will find yourself in a nice reception room furnished with a comfortable sofa and a big wardrobe. You will want to give yourself the time to decide which room to go next (i.e. kitchen, living room, bathroom or bedroom) and to choose which garment to pick from the wardrobe accordingly. Most of the time there is absolutely nothing wrong with us: we are simply not wearing the appropriate dress for the occasion. You will not feel comfortable jogging in the park in high heels, even if the weather is gorgeous! There is nothing wrong with you or with the park, it is just that you are not wearing the right gear.

So how do we get into pre-active mode? First, we want to get hold of some little tools: a small week-at-a-glance diary, a few post-it notes to stick to the inside back cover of the diary and a pen or a pencil. Make sure that you have the above with you at all times over the next few weeks. It is not difficult: ladies carry their bags with them all the time and guys have pockets or briefcases.

Then, follow the steps below:

1. When you feel the negative emotion write it down on one of the post-its in the inside back cover of your diary: write down briefly 'what' is going on and 'how' you feel about it (i.e. have received a phone call from my ex-partner – feel very sad we are no longer together).

2. Open your diary and make an appointment with yourself to deal with it. You ask yourself two questions: *when* is the appropriate time and *where* is the suitable place to deal with it? For now a ten-minute appointment would do.

3. The answer to the above question will never be 'here and now'. Whatever feelings you are dealing with, you are not a brain surgeon and nobody will die if you give yourself at least a ten-minute gap before addressing the negative emotion.

4. Number the post-it note, jot down the appointment in the diary (i.e. today at 2 pm deal with n. 3) and make sure that you remind yourself of the appointment (i.e. by setting an alarm clock or by sticking a note on your PC monitor).

5. When the time comes and you are in a proper place, for the time being just close your eyes, close your mouth, take a few deep breaths, read through your note and see how you feel. In the next steps I will show you what to do when you are there. Now, it is important that you practise first the art of making time for yourself and this is what the pre-active mode is about. I can teach you a number of useful techniques but if you don't start making time for yourself you won't be able to practise any of them.

Emotions can come our way according to two variables, which are independent of one another: intensity and urgency. So a feeling can be very intense (i.e. deep sadness, strong anger) and, at the same time, we may not feel a particular urgency to deal with it, or, on the other hand, it can be quite trivial (i.e. a bit of boredom) and we may feel that the sooner we get it out of the way the better. Practising getting yourself into pre-active mode will improve your ability of recognising your emotional states and of creating time to deal with them accordingly.

How does getting into pre-active mode work in practice? I will offer you now a real life example. Some time ago a lady came to me to receive help in dealing with an anger management problem. She was not getting along with her new boss and, at the same time, she liked her job and had a big mortgage to pay. So, leaving her job was not an option but her new manager was driving her mad and she was afraid that sooner, rather than later, she would have punched the guy in his face (incidentally she was a 6'2" tall woman).

When I introduced the different modalities and I suggested her to get into the pre-active mode during the next few days before I actually showed her what to do during our next meeting, I could see how puzzled she was by the fact that it seemed like she had nothing to do to help herself over the next week. However, when she came back for the following meeting, she had an interesting story to tell. It was the story of what had happened one day during that week.

One morning she felt like the pressure started building up at work and decided to go for a quick break. She walked down a few blocks and popped into a shop.

As she collects Swatch watches, she felt like treating herself to a new one. She was walking back to the office when she realised that she had left the watch she was wearing by the till, so she made her way back to the shop and, to try to calm herself down she kept on saying things like 'everything is going to be ok, don't worry', 'there was nobody in the shop so the assistant has surely noticed your watch by the till and he is keeping it in a safe place for you'.

However, when she got there the assistant said he did not notice anything and the watch was not there anymore! She said to me: "Tommaso, my first thought was: this cheat! He has got it and now he's pretending he knows nothing about it! I could see myself grabbing his tie and punching him with all my strength. But, at the same time, I visualised your face and you were telling me 'Please, don't do this, get into pre-active mode'. So, I shouted at the guy 'Here, this is my number, if you do find my watch call me' and stormed out of the shop. I walked into a café, got out my diary, filled in a post-it note, made an appointment with myself (that night at home looked like a proper time and place) and returned to the office."

She told me that, although she did not know what to do with her negative feeling once back home, she followed my advice of closing her eyes, closing her mouth and taking a few deep breaths. She then read what she had written on her post-it that morning and actually had a laugh as 90% of the words she used were swear words. She took comfort in toying with her collection of watches for a while and, eventually, sent an email to the company asking if they could send her the same watch she had lost.

What's so special about the above story? Well, for a start the simple fact that, because of what had happened in the shop, that could have been the day she could have displaced her anger towards her boss: she didn't. She told me that writing down her feelings, almost immediately, really helped and it also helped knowing that she had made time to deal with it. She managed to have a decent remaining part of the day at work and eventually was able to deal with it even without knowing precisely how to go about it.

So, why is getting into pre-active mode a first step in the appropriate direction? Writing down very briefly what is going on and how we feel about it is helpful because we begin an opening process whereby we allow negative feelings out of our system. Writing is also useful because it is empowering to know that we can identify and name what is happening and this helps the feeling that we can do something about it. A young lady suffering from bulimia, whom I am currently seeing, told me how good she felt about knowing that there was so much that she could do to help herself and to leave behind her past self-defeating attitude towards her emotional issues.

Creating time just for you, as you do when you make an appointment and you book it in your diary, is one of the most precious gifts you can give to yourself: there is nothing more valuable than your health and your time. Some of you may find it difficult to grant yourself permission to take care of your own issues. Sensitive and nice people are brought up to think that others always come first. I am not suggesting here that you would better mind your own business and disregard anybody else's problems. I am saying that we can, at the same time, take good care of ourselves **and** of others. Think about it for a moment. How can you really be able to be there for others and guarantee a good degree of continuity and quality in the care you offer if you don't take good care of your own issues? Do you remember what the cabin crew say when we are on a plane and about to take off? In an emergency, first adjust the oxygen mask on yourself and then help others. We can carry on being nice, friendly and supportive as much as we want and, at the same time, we can set aside a few moments during the day to deal with our issues and recharge our batteries.

Activities Box 29.

Time for your *PAL* ...
How have you dealt with your emotions so far? Have you been mostly lashing out, taking in, displacing, interrupting or daydreaming?

and for your *BIT.*
Get yourself the tools required to practise the pre-active mode and go for it!

Emotions

Seventh step
Listening to your emotional self

Now that you know how to get ready for the journey through your emotional land, thanks to the practice of getting into pre-active mode, let's see how you can move from a situation where you experience negative feelings to one where you feel happy.

The first step is to change from feeling negative emotions to being at peace with yourself and with the world. Some people find it very difficult to let themselves go with the flow and relax, even for very short periods of time. Their rational mind is constantly switched on as they try to control every behaviour and scrutinise each sensation.

This inability to de-stress affects many well-educated professionals who make a very sophisticated use of their rational resources. The other side of the coin is that they may push a bit too far and send their brains into over-drive: in such cases the fatigued and over-spinning rational mind completely takes over from the emotional one and the person gets stuck in a vicious spiral of negative automatic thoughts (i.e. panic attacks) or gets to a point where it lacks the energy to go – as a result of wasting a vast amount of resources on unnecessary activities – and shuts down most of its operating systems (i.e. breaks down), or finds it difficult to stay still, even for just five consecutive seconds.

When I ask the persons I work with for a list of relaxing activities, they usually come up with activities which provide distraction more than relaxation, such as watching the television, playing a game, going to the movies, etc. Distracting our rational mind is naturally healthy and useful and we will talk about this later when we will introduce the steps associated with the rational level. However, here we are interested in those activities that provide a connection with our emotional self.

As we have seen in the first part of this guide, the connections between our emotional brain and our body are much denser than the ones between our emotional brain and our rational brain.

Therefore, it makes sense to start by showing you, first, how to relax your body and then how to relax your mind. To do that I will teach you now two simple techniques: the Basic Body Relaxation exercise and the Insight Breathing.

Basic Body Relaxation (BBR).

Sit comfortably somewhere, loosen any tight clothing (i.e. belts, ties, bras, etc.), close your eyes and mouth and begin slowing down the pace of your breathing. Your first goal is to make sure that your breathing is slow, deep and that it provides a good supply of oxygen to your body.

If you breathe in and out through your nose, you will be able to check the pace of your breathing: a fast pace will be easily heard through the noise made by your nose, while a slow one will be totally unheard. To make sure that your breathing is deep, that is, that you are making use of the all of your respiratory system rather than just of the upper part of your chest (as we normally do) you may wish to place one of your hands on your abdomen. Place it gently, without applying any pressure, and you will be able to feel your hand going up and down as you breath deeply in and out. This will give you an awareness of how deep your are breathing and, at the same time, will result in a pleasant and soothing sensation. When your breathing is slow and deep you are also, by default, providing your body with a good supply of oxygen.

After about three minutes of the above you may now start focusing on your body. Remember that at this point you are still with your eyes and mouth closed and you are breathing slowly and deeply. Focus first on your feet. Feel them more and more relaxed as you keep on breathing in and out. Feel them increasingly heavier as you are experiencing this pleasant sensation of relaxation. Now, move gently and gradually up to your calf and do exactly the same: first feel them more and more relaxed as you keep on breathing in and out and then feel them heavier. Move gently up to each part of your body until you will have reached and totally relaxed your head.

It normally takes five minutes to carry out this exercise, so it is possible to slot it in anywhere you are (i.e. home, office, restaurant, etc.). Some of the persons I see practise the BBR in their homes' or offices' toilets, when there is no other quiet place available. I would encourage you to practice the BBR three times a day: in the morning, mid-day and in the evening.

This, naturally, in addition to the times when you would practice it as a way to get you from a negative emotional place to a positive one.

The practice of the BBR exercise has also two additional bonuses. The first is what we may call its 'expansion effect', that is, as your ability to relax improves and your experience of the exercise develops over time, you will see that you will feel relaxed for increasingly longer periods of times after your practice (i.e. you may start from feeling calm for the next 5-10 minutes and end up feeling relaxed for the next 2-3 hours). When you are there with your eyes closed, your perception of the passing time also changes. They say that how long a minute is depends on what side of the bathroom door you are on. In this case, it may feel like you have been there breathing in and out for ages and then when you open up your eyes you realise that only a few minutes have gone by.

The second is the anti-ageing effect that proper breathing has on our body in general and our skin in particular. Those who practise regularly any exercise associated with slow and deep breathing know what I am talking about and if you have ever met somebody who has been practising yoga or tai chi for a period of time you will know what I mean too. So, off you go. Don't just take my word for it. Practise the BBR and you will see for yourself.

Insight Breathing (IB).

Now that you know how to relax your body, it is time to learn how to relax your mind. The most relaxing activity we can engage in is to focus our thoughts on our breathing. We can change our mood from sad to happy in a matter of minutes, but we can only be either relaxed or distressed at any one time. Therefore, when we focus our thoughts on the very basic fact that we are breathing, we cannot, at the same time, have our mind connected with other issues.

To do that, you start by practising the BBR and when you feel your body relaxed, then, move on and ask yourself three questions.

The first question is 'What would you find most relaxing to imagine that you are breathing in and out of your body?' You may say 'What kind of question is this? I am breathing air, what else would I breathe?' You see, we do know that we are breathing air, but the point here is what would we find 'most relaxing' to imagine that we are breathing.

When you are there with your eyes closed, seated comfortably, with your body relaxed and you ask yourself the above question, you never know what answer may come up. Somebody once told me that he imagined himself seated at the bottom of a swimming pool, on one of these comfortable deck chairs, and he found it very relaxing to visualise himself breathing the 'blue' water of the pool. A lady found extremely calming the idea of breathing a bright orange 'plasmatic' substance made of some sort of 'fluid powder'. Whatever comes up, it is absolutely fine. This is your exercise and you want to make sure that you visualise something that really relaxes you and if this is simply air, that's absolutely ok, as long as you ask the question.

The second is 'What colour(s) would you associate with calm, peace and relaxation?' There surely are colours you would associate with excitement, fear or sadness. Which one(s) would you link with relaxation? If, for example, your chosen breathing medium is air and your relaxing colour is pale blue, then imagine that all the air around you is pale blue and that you are breathing in and out of your body pale blue air.

The third is 'What temperature would you associate with relaxation?' Some like it hot or warm, others prefer it cold or cool. If you are not sure you may try practising both and see which one makes you feel more relaxed.

The main thing is that, as a result of asking yourself three questions about what you are breathing, you are totally focussed on just one thing: your breathing. Therefore, you are effectively switching off your mind from the usual everyday worries and once you are there, silent, quiet, completely relaxed, physically and mentally disconnected from rational concerns, you will be able to listen to your emotional self.

It is very difficult (if not impossible) to hear a single voice speaking to us if we keep on spinning around and are in a noisy and crowded open space. But, when we create a little time for ourselves and find a conveniently quiet place, we can hear clearly the sounds and words stemming directly from our emotional self.

I have been practising the BBR and the IB for more than six years now and I would like to offer you the following tip: even when you get to the point of mastering perfectly well the sequence of physical and mental steps, do take your time to move, nicely and gently, from one step to the other.

So, for example, with practice you may be tempted to start the IB straight-away from the final step, that is imagining that you are breathing warm pale blue air. I have found it much more appropriate to keep on moving gradually in that direction, by visualising first what is it that I am breathing, and moving then onto its colour and, finally, its temperature.

The same applies to the BBR. I still find it useful to first focus on slowing down the pace of my breathing, and then to concentrate on how deep it is, rather than trying to manage both at the same time.

I would encourage you to practise the IB soon after the BBR. It may take between three and five minutes to carry out the IB, which added to the five minutes of the BBR makes a total time of eight to ten minutes.

Activities Box 30.

Time for your *PAL* ...
How have you been trying to relax so far? Have you ever tried any of the above exercises or were you mostly distracting yourself?

and for your *BIT.*
Practise the BBR and the IB three times a day.

Emotions

Eighth step
Talking to your emotional self

To make sure that you leave behind your negative feelings and consolidate your being in a peaceful place, I recommend the practice of a third exercise which I have called the 3Bs.

The 3 Breaths.

The 3Bs consists of a series of nine breaths taken soon after we end the IB exercise. It is called the 3Bs because, as you will see in a moment, there is a minor variation in what we say to ourselves during the first, second and third series of three slow and deep 'in and out' breaths.

Let's first see how you practise this technique and, then, I will tell you what is going on in your emotional self when you carry out this simple exercise.

Once you will have completed the IB, you will still be there seated comfortably with your eyes and mouth closed. Now, you say something to yourself in your mind and at the same slow pace as you are breathing in and out. Every time you breathe in, you say 'I am here'. When you breathe out, the first series of three breaths you say 'relaxed', the second series you say 'calm', the third series you say 'at peace'. In addition, only when you say 'at peace' you put a little smile on your face. The little smile fades away when you breathe in and say 'I am here' and appears again on your face when you say 'at peace'.

As you can see, it is a very simple exercise. So simple that it may make you wonder 'do we need a psychologist to come and tell us to talk to ourselves like this?' Well, we have lost so much basic wisdom, over the past 50 years, as individuals and as a society, that nowadays I don't take anything for granted when I deal with fellow human beings.

Having said that, there is a reason why I ask you to say to yourself exactly these words and precisely some words when you breathe in and others when you breathe out. Using as a reference figure 2 may help follow my explanation.

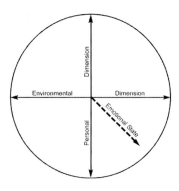

Figure 2. The Three-Dimensional Being

The circle in figure 2 represents us as human beings. In reality each of us is a full, solid body, with its three dimensions (i.e. height, width and depth). The vertical axis is our 'Personal Dimension'. It represents where we are at a given time. So, for example, when we are connected with our past, we are centred somewhere along the lower segment of this vertical dimension, while when we are associated with our wishes and desires, that is with our future, we are somewhere along the upper segment. Depending on your personal approach to life, you may see the lower segment as the metaphor for the past, the unconscious, the deeper or inner self, the soul, etc. Likewise, you may see the upper segment as representing the future, the conscious, the higher self, etc. This vertical 'Personal Dimension' (height) is our 'I am' co-ordinate.

The horizontal axis is our 'Environmental Dimension'. It represents how we relate with the world around us. So, for example, when we are emotionally connected with the things around us, with the physical environment, we are centred somewhere along the left segment, while when we are more associated with the persons around us, with the social environment, we are somewhere along the right segment. This horizontal dimension (width) is our 'here' co-ordinate.

Finally, the third dimension, the one that represents the depth co-ordinate of our being, is the one identified with our emotional state.

The first 'I am' dimension answers the question 'Who?', the second 'Here' dimension answers the question 'Where?', the third the question 'How?' So we may be sad, distressed and bored or we may be relaxed, calm and happy.

So where might we be, at a given time, within our own planet? How do we know if we are centred or we are keeping ourselves at the edges of our world?

When we experience personal distress we keep ourselves on the edges of our planet and we face outwards turning our back on all the resources, which could help us feel differently about our situation (i.e. personal resources like the awareness of where we have been or where we could be, or physical resources like what we have acquired and achieved over the years, or social resources like our friends and family).

What can we do about it, then? Well, we want to make sure that we face inwards rather than outwards and that we direct ourselves towards the centre of our planet, that is, towards a safer place.

How do we do that? We will see later how this will be achieved rationally, but now let's see how practising the 3Bs can help centre ourselves emotionally.

As we have just said, our goal is to centre ourselves. The 3Bs exercise asks you to say in your mind nine times 'I am here' as you breathe in. When you breathe in, the movement is from the external environment towards you. Most importantly, there is only one place where the 'I am' meets the 'here' and this place is the centre of our being. Therefore, every time we slowly and deeply breathe in, we are moving towards our central safer place.

At the same time, we are also breathing out that we are relaxed, calm and at peace. This gives the third co-ordinate to our position within our being, ensuring that we don't move back to the periphery of our planet and we stay centred. This time, as we breathe out, the movement is from our inner self towards the external environment. This and the fact that we put a little smile on our face, serves like a training activity to make sure that when the exercise is over, we can go back to our every day life *really* feeling relaxed, calm and at peace.

I hope the above makes sense to you, but, even if it doesn't, don't worry.

Emotional techniques are not supposed to make sense rationally (it would be a disaster if the rational techniques would not make sense logically!) they are meant to nurture your emotional self.

The practise of the 3Bs does not take more than a couple of minutes, which added to the eight to ten minutes of the BBR + IB exercises gives a total of ten to twelve minutes. Now, as you can see, I am not asking you to leave your jobs, shave your heads, wear orange robes and sandals and start singing 'Hare Krsna, hare, hare...' down the street. I am also not asking you to practise lengthy and complicated exercises, which would occupy considerable parts of your day.

If you are motivated to take care of yourself and look after your emotional well-being, a ten-minute practice, two or three times a day, is something that can easily be fitted into even the busiest daily schedules.

Activities Box 31.

Time for your *PAL* ...
Write down your thoughts about how differently you may deal with a given situation or event, when you are stressed and angry or you are calm and relaxed.

and for your *BIT.*
Practise the 3Bs regularly (ideally three times a day, soon after the BBR and the IB).

Emotions

Ninth step
Dealing with negative feelings

Now that you know how to take yourself from a place where you experience negative feelings to another where you feel calm and relaxed, let's see how to help you connect with strong positive emotions. Before we do that, however, I would like to remind you that getting to a happy emotional state does not represent the end of your person care journey, rather it is just a step forward in the appropriate direction. When you disconnect from negative emotions to make peace with yourself and connect with positive ones, you are unplugging and re-plugging your emotional system, thus resetting your emotional self.

As illustrated in figure 3, the next steps will show you how to deal with your issues by leading you across Leonardo's Bridge, the bridge of Creativity and Reason, to the HUH land (Healthy, Useful and Helpful). This is a place where you will be able to connect with all your resources and where you will find some answers to your questions. You will explore the territory of HUH during the rational component part of your journey. First, let's get started with the final step of the emotional component.

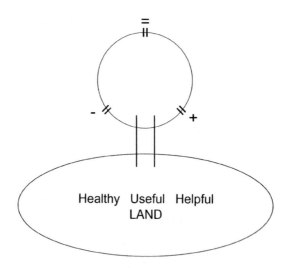

Figure 3. The first level of the IPC Process

The Positive Association (PA).

This technique has two main goals: to make sure that you strongly connect with a happy feeling and to remain associated with that positive emotion for a while. To use a simple metaphor: imagine that you are on holiday. You are seated on a boat and you are exploring the coastline and the surrounding sea. The sea is crystal clear and though you know that it is 60 or 70 meters deep, it looks like it is just 20 meters deep.

You notice something glistening at the bottom of the sea: it is a beautiful pearl. Your goal is to dive down there, catch the pearl and bring it back to the surface with you. Naturally, it would be appropriate to go down and, most importantly, to come up gently and gradually. Divers know that you are required to have a few compensation breaks on your way back to the surface to help the body re-adjust to the different pressures.

How do you practise the PA? First of all, you begin by practising the BBR, the IB and the 3Bs. When you feel you are in a much calmer place, then you stay there with your eyes closed and start the PA.

The Positive Association exercise consists of a number of steps. You go through these steps as you go down and you take the same steps backwards when you return. One thing I am telling you now, so that I won't repeat myself later, is that in between each step you are required to have your 'decompression times' in the form of breathing breaks.

So, to ensure that you go down and come back gradually, you take a few slow and deep breaths in between each step, to allow you the opportunity to fully connect with that particular step and to make sure that you move from one step to the next gently and gradually. How many you take is up to you. That depends on the time at your disposal.

If you were to take five deep breaths in between each step, the whole exercise would last approximately 15 minutes. If you have more time to enjoy this pleasurable exercise, you may take longer breaks.

Now, let's introduce the steps.

1. Think of a very happy memory, or a very happy fantasy.

2. Identify the happiest part/scene of the above memory or fantasy.

3. Visualise on your inner screen the happiest part/scene. It doesn't matter if your visualisation is in black and white, colour or 3D, as long as you have a strong feeling that you can clearly see the picture.

4. Imagine you are in a cinema and you are seeing a movie. First, the picture you have just visualised becomes as big as a movie screen (quantitative change) and, then, starts getting in motion, like you were watching a real movie (qualitative change). You are starring in this movie and you can see yourself living or re-living this very happy moment.

5. Step in the movie. Now you are not able to see yourself living or re-living the moment, you *are* living or re-living it. So, for example, let's assume that your fantasy is to lay down on a golden sandy beach, with the sun shining and a turquoise sea only a few feet away. In the previous step – the cinema situation – you could see yourself lying down and enjoying the holiday, while in this step you can actually feel the sun on your skin and smell the sea breeze.

6. At this moment in time, you will feel very happy. Now, that you have found your 'pearl' it is time to grab it with both hands. So, ask yourself 'Which part of my body feels happiest now?' or 'Where is the centre of my happiness?' You don't want to analyse yourself now, this is meant to be a very straightforward question, which attracts a simple and intuitive answer. Some people say 'the centre of my forehead', other 'my neck' or 'my tummy' or 'my hands'. There aren't right or wrong answers: just say in your mind what comes up first.

7. Spread this pleasant sensation of happiness all over your body now, nicely and gently. Make sure that you don't leave any part of your body out. So, for example, if your centre was your abdomen, start by spreading the pleasurable sensation of happiness all the way down to your feet and then move up, right up to the top of your head or vice versa, as you like. How do you spread your sensation of happiness throughout your body? Some people associate happiness with a gentle touch and they imagine that a feather, a leaf or a small hand is touching them. Others imagine an energy field or a liquid expanding all over their body. In one case the energy field was white and the liquid was orange. You may wish to try any of the above or find something different.

Once the pleasurable sensation of happiness has been spread all over your body, it is time to go back.

However, as you move backwards you don't want to lose what you have achieved, you want to bring your 'pearl' back to the surface.

So, you do go through the same steps backwards, but with a very important difference: every time you move from one step to the next you say to yourself: 'I am moving backwards now **and**, at the same time, I am keeping this nice (or 'pleasurable', as you prefer) sensation of happiness spread all over my body' and off you go to the next step.

You say to yourself the same thing every time you are moving backwards: as a result, when you open your eyes, the nice sensation of happiness will still be there spread all over your body.

The Breathing Visualisation Exercise (BVE).

The purpose of this technique is to enable you to deal appropriately with potentially stressful events or difficult situations that you know you will face in the near future. I suggest you practise it, once or twice a day, in the period of time before the event.

The technique consists of four consecutive steps:

a) first, sit somewhere comfortably and practise for a few minutes the Basic Body Relaxation (BBR);

b) then, keeping your eyes closed, you visualise yourself doing all the things that you would normally do just before the event, in a very relaxed fashion (i.e. if you are concerned about an exam or a job presentation scheduled for 10 am, you see yourself waking up, having breakfast, showering, getting dressed, going out, walking into your office and sitting at your desk); this is the 'before step';

c) now, you visualise yourself going through the event in a very relaxed, comfortable and confident manner; this is the 'during step';

d) finally, you congratulate yourself for the way you have handled the event and, if this is the case, you consider how you can further improve your behaviour or performance; this is the 'after step'.

How can this technique help you? Well, it utilises the wonderful power of our brain to make associations.

Normally, we would associate an event with a sensation or feeling, which could be pleasant or unpleasant (i.e. a piece of music or a song may remind you of your first love or your first slow dance, thus eliciting a pleasant response; or a loud noise may trigger the memory of a car crash).

This time, we use the same power but the other way around: that is, we associate a preceding mood with a current event, because the practice of the BVE will train your brain to associate being calm, comfortable and relaxed when going through a particular event.

A tip I would suggest is that you include in the 'before step' a routine you are very familiar with, something that you know will happen before the event and that you will find easy to visualise: getting off to a good start can significantly improve the efficacy of this technique!

I could offer you plenty of examples on how practising the BVE has helped many persons I have seen: we go from panic attacks caused by certain situations (i.e. travelling by tube or by plane, or taking a lift), to events such as exams, functions and presentations.

The first which springs to mind is the case of a bright and talented young professional who was holding back his career because of his fear of speaking in public. This would prevent him from giving presentations which would have dramatically improved his professional standing within his company.

He made the best possible use, through regular practice, of all three steps of the BVE technique visualising himself, first, going through the morning routine at home in a very relaxed fashion; then, dealing with a presentation in a calm and confident manner; finally, congratulating himself, while, at the same time, considering how he could have improved his performance, the next time around.

This latter step provided a useful feedback. Given that one of the main triggers for his lack of confidence was the fear of being asked questions he would not know the answer to – though he was very knowledgeable in his area of expertise, he introduced, at the very start of his presentation, an initial statement where he would say:

"Thank you for giving me the opportunity to present this (indicating here the topic). I would welcome your questions and requests for further information. In the likely event (smiling) I would not know the answer to your questions, at present, here are my contact details (he would either write on the flip chart his phone number and email address, or have the details indicated on the presentation info-pack), please feel free to get in touch and I will get back to you."

By saying the above, he was then able to begin the presentation in a much more relaxed and confident manner.

Activities Box 32.

Time for your *PAL* ...
Think about how you would connect with happy feelings in the past and note down similarities and differences.

and for your *BIT.*
Practise the PA and the BVE regularly, at least once a week. Learning how to take care of yourself is just like learning a language (in this case, the language of your emotional self). You'll never know when you will be needing them and if you don't practise, you won't be able to use them, when the occasion arises.

Chapter 9

Thoughts

*"Good-humoured patience is necessary
with mischievous children and your own mind."*

Robert Aitkin Roshi (1)

Tenth step
Exploring the association between thought and language

If I could open a tiny window in people's heads and spring-clean away their emotional ghosts and rational worries in just 2 minutes, I would have a 20-mile long queue outside my office, day and night, all year around. In reality, I am not able to do that myself, but I can teach you how to do it by yourself in the next few steps.

So, in the end, everybody will be happy: me, because I am helping you out and you, because you will learn how to take care of yourself.

Now, let's walk on Leonardo's Bridge, the bridge of Creativity and Reason, and get from the Emotional Land to the Healthy, Useful and Helpful country. You will learn three different ways of approaching your concerns, as you walk on Leonardo (the language point, the 3As and the slide show technique) which make up the next three steps of our journey.

Then, once we will have arrived in the HUH country, we will get to the root of your issues by talking about your dimensions (intrapersonal, personal and interpersonal), your time perspectives (past, present and future) and the emerging problems of relapse management (how to stay on the healthy, useful and helpful track).

The Fight or Flight Response.

The Language Point is about talking to ourselves and to others in a healthy and helpful way. Before I show you how to do that, it is important to appreciate how unhealthy and self-defeating are some common expressions we use in our everyday life and why it would be appropriate to replace them with useful ones. In order to understand the extent of the damage we cause to our system, let's, therefore, first clarify what the 'fight or flight response' is and why it does matter.

In the early 1960s, the American physician Walter Cannon introduced the concept of the 'fight or flight response' when referring to the following basic human biological process and associated behaviour. When we are confronted with a dangerous and potentially life threatening situation, our body gets ready to fight or flee. It does that by increasing our heart beat, raising our blood pressure, pumping blood to the appropriate muscles and releasing adrenal hormones. After the fight or the run, as a result of having fought or fled, our body gets back to its natural balance (i.e. slower heart beat and breathing pace).

Now, in the old days, a few hundred thousand years ago, humans were faced with the choice of fighting or fleeing for a number of very simple and basic reasons (predators, hostile tribes, shortage of food supply or routine hunting) and they had plenty of opportunities to elicit the biological response and to get back to a position of balance after the fight or the run. What about us?

Whether you like it or not, we haven't changed much over the past few hundred thousand years, apart from a bit of body hair left behind in our caves (we don't need it anymore in our comfortable and heated homes). This means that when we **perceive** a situation, or a life's event as threatening, we still have the same biological response and still need to release the energy produced and the tension accumulated in an appropriate way. The point is, can we respond to our contemporary stressors like our ancestors, by fighting or fleeing?

If you are attending a meeting where the closure of your company's business is being discussed, with the prospect of many employees – including yourself – being made redundant in the near future, would you start punching and kicking the hell out of your managers or would you jump and run away?

If you left it to the very last day and the very last moment to pay a bill and you had the brilliant idea of going down to the post office or the bank during your lunch break because the rest of the day you are fully booked and you find a very long queue, would you start knocking down all the people in front of you or would you flee the scene?

As you can see, although we do experience very high levels of stress, as a result of how we perceive our reality, nowadays we find it more difficult to release that energy and tension in such a way that it would not harm anybody, including ourselves. So, some people *explode* turning against their fellow humans verbally (i.e. shouting, insulting), mentally (hating, plotting), or physically (smashing furniture, slapping, punching), while others *implode* turning against themselves (depression, compulsive behaviours, anxiety attacks, eating disorders).

As Kathleen Malley-Morrison notes:
"Unfortunately, we have not advanced very far in teaching our children alternatives to fighting and fleeing when they feel threatened, so there is still an awful lot of fighting going on...However, despite the strong human propensity for aggression, we also know that violence is not inevitable. Human beings are capable of dealing with threats, managing anger, and responding to frustration in non-violent ways...so there's hope." (2)

Now that we know what is going on, what can we do about it? Well, we can, on the one hand, learn how to avoid putting pressure on ourselves, to minimise the release of stress hormones, and, on the other, we can learn how to release appropriately the tension once it is already there.

The Language Point.

There are two categories of words that would be appropriate to delete from our vocabulary: the imperatives and the self-defeating. The imperatives are expressions like: *I must, I should, I have to, I ought to, this is urgent.* Every time we say them, we place a weight on our shoulder. Every time we pronounce them we colour in a particular way our reality, perceiving life's events not just as they are, but in a darker and more powerful light. This triggers a fight or flight biological response with all the consequences seen above.

If you are in the habit of using imperatives on a daily basis, imagine how much damage this has caused to your system – that is, to your physiological, emotional and rational components, as a whole – over the past few years.

Self-defeating words are expressions like: *I cannot* and *I need*. Every time we say them we corner ourselves facing a huge wall of our own making. If you cannot, you cannot, what else can you do? If you need, you need, how else can you go about it? Do you see how dis-empowering these expressions are? If you are normally using these words, do you see how much damage this has caused to your self-esteem, day after day, week after week, over the past few years?

We use self-defeating words also when we repeatedly talk about our alleged illnesses, when we say "I am depressed", "I am hopeless", "I feel so low". As Italian psychiatrist, Raffaele Morelli puts it: *"In so doing, we are actually creating the illness, rather than dealing with it!" (3)*

How can we rephrase imperatives and self-defeating expressions?

Let's start from the imperatives. You may use them on two occasions: personal life or professional life's events. If you are using them to refer to personal life events (i.e. I must go to the gym, I have to eat healthily, etc.), you are advised to replace them with preferences (i.e. I would like to, I would love to, it would be great, it would be interesting, it would be useful).

As a practical example, I offer you the experience of a young lady who came to me complaining of her dissatisfaction with her body. She had used comfort eating as a way of addressing her emotional issues and, as a result, she had put on considerable weight, which was now causing added distress. Every morning she would have her exercise-bag ready for the gym and every morning she would say to herself, literally, 'come on now, you stupid bitch, you must go to the gym' or 'you silly cow, today there are no excuses, you have to go to the gym'. Bearing in mind that the gym was located in the basement of her office building and that the fees were subsidised by her company, it really looked like it would have been so easy for her to go, so why didn't she manage to get there?

Well, now you too are aware of how there were two powerful forces in action here. The first was the reaction caused by her using imperatives in an attempt to convince herself to go to the gym. The imperatives caused a lot of pressure, which in her case easily teamed up with anxiety. Humans are pleasure seeking creatures and having a choice, we would rather pass on something associated with anxiety and procrastinate than engage with it, and that's what she did.

The second was the reaction caused by her bad-mouthing herself. The inner adult was reproaching the inner child too forcefully and the resulting reaction was equally powerful. Imagine you are standing still and, at the same time, one person is pulling your right arm and another one is pulling your left arm, which way would you go? You are stuck there, not free to move either way and, in the process, this also hurts. That was exactly the place where this lady was when she came to see me.

My answer was simple and clear: stop fighting with yourself. It's a war lost from the start and, though it may look like you are winning a few battles now and then, in the end there will be no winners and only one loser: you. How to go about it, then? Make peace with yourself. Treat yourself nicely, gently and with respect. Listen to your inner adult and, at the same time, let your inner child play. I introduced her to the behavioural self-help steps and guided her through my person care process.

How did it go with the gym? As soon as she replaced imperatives with 'I enjoy going to the gym' or 'I would like to go to the gym, because it makes me feel better' she started exercising regularly for not less than three times a week.

How do you rephrase imperatives when you apply them to work situations? Here, of course, the use of preferences does not seem appropriate. In real life most people – though they may like their jobs and find them interesting or stimulating – are not really in love with their profession and having a choice they would rather do something else with their time. So, let's use as an example a typical sentence, which can be easily adapted to your own circumstances: 'I must complete this report by the end of the week.'

First, let's note how unhealthy the above sentence is. When we use the expression 'I must' not only may we trigger the fight or flight biological response, whose associated natural behaviours would clash with our professional duty, but we also start off by putting ourselves in a victim situation. 'I must...poor me...this is unfair...why should I?' The above sentence allows no boundaries between who we are, as persons, what we do for a living, at this given time in our life, and the task in hand. This means that we totally identify ourselves – and our sense of self-worth – with the job we do and how we perform in this specific task.

This way, if we perform 7 out of 10, we are more likely to feel unhappy or concerned about not having reached a full result than to be happy about having achieved 7. We are more than what we do for a living during a given time of our life and much more than a single – though very important – task. When we talk to ourselves like this, we create a black hole, which inevitably sucks in who we are and the very reasons why we are doing what we are doing with our life.

The likely consequence of talking like that will be to procrastinate and wait until the very last moment to get the report done, which naturally does not help improve the quality of our work. In such cases, we may use virtually anything to reduce the anxiety caused by the way we perceive our situation ('I must...') and we may end up tiding up a desk which had not been given any attention for the past three years and could have waited, at least, a few more weeks, or sorting computer files that had never attracted our attention since their original creation.

Let's see how just some minor but significant changes can turn an unhealthy sentence into a helpful one. I would like you to rephrase the sentence like this: 'I know that my professional goal (or objective) is to complete this report by the end of the week'.

Noticed the differences? Well, first of all, you are not saying 'I must' you are saying 'I know'. In your mind this is the equivalent of walking upright rather than walking with a heavy weight on your shoulders or dragging around an iron ball chained to your ankle.

When you say 'I know' you associate yourself with your resources, with all that you know and studied or trained for, rather than connecting with your doubts and fears. Then you say 'that my professional goal is to...', and this helps you see the event for what it really is: that you are a person who has decided to carry out a given profession which, in turn, requires you to complete a specific task. This allows the creation of healthy boundaries between who you are and what you do for a living, which are essential for building and keeping up your self-esteem.

If you talked to yourself like this you are more likely to carry out your given task and also more likely to perform better. You are also more likely to contribute to the improvement of your work procedures or environment, because you will be able to put forward sound reasons to justify the changes and motivate your colleagues and managers.

How do we rephrase self-defeating expressions like 'I cannot' and 'I need'?

Well, the latter can be rephrased exactly like you do with the imperatives. The former, instead, can be replaced by using the relevant adjective. You see, each time we say 'I cannot', we corner ourselves into a situation where there is no way out but retreating. Imagine yourself facing the corner of your room and walking towards it. At some point you will stop, otherwise you will bang your head on the wall. If you go right or left, you hit the wall, so the only way out is going backwards. This is exactly what happens in your mind when you say 'I cannot'. You take your brain to a very frustrating place. The answer is: say what you mean. In reality, 99.9% of the time you mean:

I find this extremely difficult, or
I find this very difficult, or
I find this quite difficult, or
I find this fairly difficult, or
I find this difficult.

The difference is that when you use any of the above, from the most powerful ('extremely') to the less forceful (just difficult), you are not cornering your brain and your mind will be more likely to suggest ways to go around or beneath your hurdle.

I could give you many examples of how practising the language point has improved the life of many of the persons I have seen over the past five years. The first case that springs to mind, which is also the last in chronological order, is that of a young lady suffering from bulimia whose comment was: *"Tommaso, look, when I first heard you talking about this I thought 'what a nonsense... this is bullshit... I don't believe I am here listening to this man'. Then I decided to take your word for it, after all I had nothing to lose and there was no harm in trying, if only to come back to you in two weeks' time and tell you in your face what crap this whole thing was. But, now...I don't know how to put this...I believe this thing actually works. I know it's early days but I feel that there is so much I can do to help myself, whereas in the past I would carry on thinking only about all the things I could not do".*

My tips about how to go about practising the language point are: the sooner you start practising the language point the better. However, go with the flow and don't put pressure on yourself. It will take some time for you to re-adjust to a new healthy way of talking to yourself and to others, don't be in a hurry.

When you realise that you have just used an imperative or a self-defeating word, don't beat yourself up. To the contrary, congratulate yourself for having been able to spot the difference and rephrase the expression. You are not competing against someone else. Do not compete against yourself.

I have started practising the language point six years ago and now, in those rare occasions when an unhealthy word like 'I need' or 'I cannot' slips through, first, I realise how just the sound of it clashes with my internal state, then I spontaneously smile, and, finally, I rephrase it saying what I mean.

Activities Box 33.

Time for your *PAL* …
Think about the fight and flight response. What are the similarities and differences that you find between our life as humans a few hundred thousand years ago and now.

and for your *BIT.*
Start practising the language point.

Thoughts

Eleventh step
Dealing with negative thoughts

The second exercise we meet, as we keep on walking on Leonardo's Bridge, is **the 3As**, which has been created for the purpose of helping you deal with negative thoughts. The three As stand for:

- ✓ Acknowledgement
- ✓ Awareness
- ✓ Action

First, let's see what meaning we attach to the above words and I will, then, give you an example of how this exercise has been applied to a real life situation. Please note that, where possible, I would recommend carrying out this exercise in writing.

The **acknowledgement** step answers the question 'what is this all about?' This step gives you the opportunity to recollect precisely what has triggered your negative thinking (i.e. an abusive phone call from an ex-partner, an inappropriate comment from a colleague, the sudden illness of a dear friend, etc.).

I have found in my professional experience that persons at times sink deep down into a spiral of negative thoughts as a result of something that they have genuinely misheard, misinterpreted or misconstrued. In such instances, it was not a case of actually dealing with a difficult or problematic negative event, rather it was about acknowledging that our misperception of what happened at that time had tricked us into believing that we heard something when something else had been said.

I recommend going through the 3As steps in writing, whenever possible, as this helps clarify the issues. Naturally, the best way to go about this step would be to ask our interlocutor to clarify their point (i.e. 'did I hear you correctly when you said...'). When this is not feasible, going back to notes taken at the time may help, or reading again the letter or email that caused our distress in the first place.

Failing all of the above, just write down what you think has happened – now that you are gently walking on Leonardo's Bridge and you are calm and relaxed. It is important to note that what you are doing here is not analysing yourself or the situation, but, rather, just observing it.

The **awareness** step answers, in three ways, the question 'why has this happened?' In the English language the terms *acknowledgement* and *awareness* may at times be used as synonyms. In their IPC connotations, they have a different meaning: the awareness step is deeper and more connected with higher rational processes than the initial acknowledgment one. Here you ask yourself three questions:

> ➤ *Why do I think this has happened?*
> This is your own interpretation of the event.

> ➤ *What a third party thinks about what has happened? (if nobody else was present at the time or you don't feel it would be appropriate to ask, what a camera would have seen?)*
> This is the account provided by a friend or a colleague, or an explanation based on your essential description (just like a camera was filming the event).

> ➤ *Why would I do or say something like that, if I were this person?*
> This is you focussing on the person who has caused you distress and stepping in their shoes.

The **action** step answers to the question 'how to go about this?'

In real life, most of us, not only don't give ourselves the chance to relax and calm down, like we suggest doing as you go through a few minutes' practice of the emotional level exercises, but also jump straightaway from thinking a negative thought to performing their (explosive or implosive) response in a matter of seconds.

It goes without saying that such actions – or reactions – do not adequately address the issue and, in most cases, actually end up making things worse. If we follow the IPC steps and we approach our issues not earlier than when we are walking on Leonardo's Bridge, things can be different, as the following case illustrates.

A young woman came to me complaining about her difficult work situation. She was a dark-haired, tall, very good looking and well-educated Anglo-French lady. She had been working for the same multinational company for a number of years and up to that moment she had been enjoying her job as a personal assistant to one of the directors of the London office. Her job was well paid and, most importantly, her working time gave her the opportunity to attend a part-time Master degree programme in Business Administration.

She had a very good relationship with her boss, who would value her opinion and discussed regularly work issues with her. Unfortunately, her boss decided to take an early retirement and go back to his country and the new one did not seem to connect with her at all. Her professional situation had become such a source of distress that she had thought of resigning from her position. I was her last chance to try to do something about it.

The core of the problem was essentially the way the new boss was treating her. The previous director was a middle-aged Spanish gentleman with impeccable manners and a fine sense of humour, the new one was a young English guy whom she could hardly see in person, as he would get into work before her, leave after her and, above all, communicate with her mostly through internal emails.

The way he gave her directives was driving her nuts: she would find folders piled up on her desk in the morning with brief but detailed instructions typed on an A4 sheet of paper. She said "that jerk does not even have the decency to use the fucking phone!". There was none of the niceties and warm interactions she had with the previous boss and none of the professional discussion where she felt that her experience in the role and her intellectual abilities were valued and utilised. She suddenly felt downgraded to a role of typist she had never performed even during the early days of her employment with the company.

We agreed to get together for a couple of intensive meetings where I would show her how to take care of her physiological and emotional levels and then once on Leonardo's Bridge, we would work gradually, step by step, through the rational level exercises. When it was time for her to practise the 3As, she offered the following feedback.

Acknowledgment.
My boss is an arrogant public school boy.

Awareness.

First why (what did she think herself).
*He looks down on me because I am not English (*she perceived herself more as French*) and because he is a bastard of a man and I am a woman.*

Second why (what did a colleague think of the situation).
The personal assistant to the other director, who shared her large office with her and whose desk was right opposite hers said: "*You may not be aware of the fact that you may come across as a woman with a strong personality and that man looks a bit shy to me. He also seems to be quite young. I bet he comes straight out of University and has had not much practical professional experience, so that's why he is probably avoiding contact with you: he may be afraid of displaying his weaknesses.*"

Third why (what did she think he was thinking).
She is just a secretary, who cares? I have far more important things to do than wasting time with her, or trying to be nice to her.

When I asked her to comment on the exercise, she said: "*Well, as you know before I practised the 3As I thought I had no option but to leave the job. I wrote down in the first why of the awareness step very much what I thought of this guy.*
Then, when I listened to what my colleague had to say – to get on board the second why – something clicked in the back of my mind. I mean, I was still thinking that he was a jerk, but there could have been one chance in a million that my colleague was right.
*Up to that moment, my reaction had been to keep it to myself. So, although we have the tradition of ending the working week by meeting down the pub on Friday evenings, I had not been down there since the new director arrived because I just wanted to avoid a big argument or a fight. But, once I felt on your bridge (*Leonardo's Bridge*) and after practising the 3As, something clicked in me and I decided to go down the pub last Friday and check this guy out for myself.*
From the very first moments I could see my colleague had been right about him. He was nice and very shy and when I got close enough for a one-to-one chat I asked him about his previous working experiences. That was his first important job and before he had been working as a researcher for his university.

At that point, I took the courage to ask why he was communicating with me as he was and I also told him that his behaviour seemed a bit odd to me. He apologised and openly confessed that he didn't mean to be rude and to diminish my role. It was just that he wanted to do his best and this was the first big opportunity he had to show his skills. That's why he would get into work very early in the morning and leave quite late. He wanted to make sure that everything was well organised and planned for the day ahead and he thought that by also organising my work load for me, by sorting out my folders and leaving me written notes, he was actually making my life easier".

The rest of the story goes that from that point on, their relationship improved as she felt almost like mothering this young chap in his new important job and he began asking her for her opinion on professional matters, as well as tips on how to improve his dress sense.

The 3As is a simple exercise and not a magical formula. Different techniques work differently for different persons. However, I believe that small changes can make a big difference. This is even more true when the small changes we apply to how we perceive ourselves and the world around us are introduced nicely and gradually, and at the appropriate time.

Activities Box 34.

Time for your *PAL* …
Think about the 3As. How have you been dealing with your negative thoughts so far and what changes does this exercise introduce in the way you appraise an event?

and for your *BIT.*
Start practising the 3As.

Thoughts

Twelfth step
Turning your thought processes into resources

The last and, probably, the most important exercise we learn during our walk on Leonardo's Bridge is the Slide Show Technique (SST). The goal of the SST is to help you re-process your thoughts in a healthy, useful and helpful way by turning them into resources.

Up to this point you have been storing the incoming information in two different containers, one for the positive and one for the negative thoughts. The downside of this way of processing and storing thoughts lies in the fact that sooner or later the two containers (especially the negative one) become full and than we hear persons say 'I have had enough' or 'I can't take this anymore' or 'this is too much for me'.

We may suffer even more when the negative container becomes full gradually, almost subtly, because the pain and confusion we experience catch us by surprise and because we find it difficult to grasp how such a minor thing (the straw that broke the camel's back) can trigger such a response. Truth is, we don't appreciate how the problem does not lie with the final little negative thought, but with the thousands we had previously allowed to sink in.

What can we do about this? We can leave the hardware as it is and take care of upgrading the software by downloading a new application: the SST. Practising the SST will change the way you process your thoughts and turn all of them, both negative and positive, into precious resources. The Language Point has shown you how to prevent placing unnecessary pressure on yourself.

The 3As has provided you with a simple strategy to ensure that you don't make a mountain out of a molehill. The Slide Show Technique will enable you to re-process all the rubbish already stored in your system and, at the same time, will help you change the processing system itself, making sure that you don't keep on storing rubbish in the future.

Now, let me ask you just one question, before I show you how to go about the SST. When does your new day start? I don't mean this in an existential philosophical way. I mean, a normal, ordinary day.

When you get up in the morning? It may look like it, but no...try again. When you wake up? Nope. When you have your breakfast? Nei. When you have your shower? Niet. When you get dressed and walk out of your house? Ohi. When you get into your office? Nein. Well, I would stop here, as I don't know any other way of saying 'no'.

The answer is: you start a new day immediately after you have closed the day before. Now, how many of you manage to close your day? Bear in mind that there are three important components to ourselves (physiological, emotional and rational) and you want to reset all three of them. If you don't reset your system by appropriately closing the previous day, you will not be able to start a new day: you will be simply carrying on the day (and week, and month, and year) before. That's why we come to a point when we say 'I have had enough!'

So, for example, when you have a late supper (with or without lots of drinks) and then you plunge into bed without allowing enough time for digesting your food, you are very likely to have poor sleep, get up in the morning not feeling rested (and maybe not even wanting to leave the bed!) and with a foul taste in your mouth. You are very likely to skip breakfast and end up at work like a zombie: your stomach empty, your mind in bed and your body wandering around the office. This is how you do not start your new day, but, rather, carry your previous one forward, physiologically.

The same applies when you don't make peace with yourself, emotionally, (remember the BBR, IB and 3BS exercises?) and carry forward emotional material belonging to one day to the next, like sweeping under the carpet a little dust every day until the day when you trip, fall over and hit your head as a result of the big bumps you have created under the carpet.

The same also applies when you don't take the time to reflect on your rational concerns and you create monsters of Worry out of negative thoughts not addressed at the appropriate time.

So, this is my point: to deal appropriately with our issues we want to make sure that we close our day, every day, thus resetting the whole of our system by allowing our brain to carry out its maintenance job and take care of our physiological hitches, emotional issues and rational concerns.

Now, let's first see how to practise this exercise and then we will add some final comments.

The Slide Show Technique (SST).

It would be useful to practise a bit of BBR and IB before starting the SST. When you find yourself seated comfortably somewhere with your eyes closed and you become aware of your state of relaxation, you may start taking the following steps:

1. Think about a slide show and imagine how you would like to create yours. For example, are your slides coming in your visual field from the right and going out to the left or the other way around, or perhaps you prefer visualising them coming in from the top or the bottom, or flashing in and out – like the slides in a powerpoint presentation. Once you have decided your chosen motion you can move to the next step.

2. Ask yourself 'has anything meaningful happened today?' If nothing comes up, you practise the 3Bs and you are done. If more items come up, you just pick one of them and work through it, as indicated below.

3. Allow the item to come in your visual field, like a slide in a slide show. Visualise it as clearly as possible. It doesn't matter if the slide is in black & white, colour or 3D, as long as you have a clear visualisation any format is fine.

4. Ask yourself how do you feel about this event? Is this item positive (i.e. a colleague paying you a compliment) or negative (i.e. a difficult meeting with a former friend).

5. Now you want to consolidate your appreciation of this event as positive or negative by 'framing' it as positive or negative. You can do this by visualising yourself writing on the top of the slide with a pen or with your finger a plus (+),or a minus (-) sign, or writing 'positive' or 'negative', or using a colour which, like an aura, goes around the slide (i.e. there was

167

a lady who would visualise a tubular neon sign going around the slide and the sign turned black for negative and orange for positive).

6. Ask yourself 'what can I learn from this?' Please note that this question is not future oriented. It is a simple question designed, among other things, to make sure that you are able to make peace with yourself and reset your system. So, we are not asking the question to elicit any deep philosophical revelation or to find the solution to one of the endemic problems afflicting humanity. Just go with the flow, be happy with everything you get with this exercise and don't vet what your system is bringing up to the surface (i.e. don't say things like "this item is too trivial to be worked through let's fish another one", or "this answer is too simple let's think of something more intelligent"). Humans have developed on this planet thanks to their extraordinary capacity to make sense of things and learn from them. So, don't worry. Be there, calm and relaxed, and you will see that one or more answers will come to you.

7. Now that you know that you have learnt something from this particular positive or negative event, it is time to reframe it as a learning experience. To do that say to yourself in your mind "now that I have learnt this (and you name what you have learnt) this event has become a learning experience" and you consolidate this by visualising yourself first brushing off the previous positive or negative framing and then writing on the top of your slide either a symbol of your choice (i.e. a diamond, a star, an asterisk, etc.) if you used a symbol (+ or -) to frame the slide before, or if you wrote 'positive' or 'negative' you can now write 'learning experience' on its top. If you used a colour around the slide, you can now choose a new colour (the lady of the example before had her neon sign turning green).

8. The event you have been dealing with has become a learning experience. It is not a positive or negative item anymore. Now that you have washed away its unhealthy charge and unhelpful connotation you can let it slide away from your visual field and into your storage system. You can go back and see if there is any other meaningful thing, which has happened during the day, and work through it the same way.

So, what happened to the item when you let it go? It is not negative anymore, so it won't go in the negative container and it is not positive anymore, so it won't go in the positive container.

Truth is, our brain has already a nice chest of drawers ready for it, where items are stored by topics rather than by charge and connotation. This is the software upgrade I was referring to at the beginning of this step. Your system had been ready for it since birth, but you had never used this advanced option so far. There are drawers for all sorts of items and topics. The beautiful thing is: topics will never come back from the past to haunt you – as negative thoughts, like ghosts, can do – topics are resources that will spring to mind only to make you feel better.

What happens to the material already stored in our containers? As I said, your brain will recognise immediately that you are using its most advanced application and, as you keep on practising the SST every day, it will gradually convert items previously stored in the bins into topics and store them in the relevant drawer.

I warmly recommend that you practise the SST on a daily basis. When? Whenever it suits you. Some practise as soon as they are back at home in the evening, some after supper or before going to bed, others on the train as they commute back home from work.

What happens if you forget or skip one day? Nothing serious really. It is easier and healthier to deal with your issues on a daily basis. The following day you will work on two days rather than one.

When you get into the habit of closing your day, every day, wonderful little things will happen to you and I'm talking about those little things that make your life worth living.

Also, the next time life throws at you something unpleasant, you are more likely to say "hum, hang on a moment, I have been here before and I know what to do..." making use of your experience and connecting with your rational resources, rather than sinking in a downward negative spiral and saying "oh, dear here it goes again...how can I go about it now...why is this happening to me now? ...it's all happening now, am I cursed, or something?"

At this point you may ask "Look, we can see why it would be useful to get rid of the negative container, but why do you want to get rid of the positive one too? Wouldn't it be nice to keep the positive bin?

You see this is when we face the transition from theory to practice. Useful theories help us improve our real life and the old two-bins system is not doing us any favour. I have seen persons suffering considerable psychological pain as a result of having their positive bins filled up. How is this possible?

These persons had lost the capacity to look forward, the drive to live their lives because they were living in their past, all immersed in cuddling their happy memories. They began isolating themselves from friends and family and fell first into a state of pleasurable numbness, then into depression and finally into a psychotic condition where they were not able to tell anymore which dimension was real, the one they had in their mind or the one they had around them. Their positive bin had become a powerful magnet, which – just like a black hole – was sucking in their vital energy, disconnecting these persons from their present and future.

When we practise the SST we don't simply get rid of the positive bin, we convert it into a precious and more advanced resource system, which we will be using as a helpful ally throughout our life.

As Italian psychiatrist, Raffaele Morelli, notes: *"Thoughts are still, whereas the life forces within us constantly flow."* (4)

The SST helps you reprocess your thoughts and free yourself from their unhealthy stillness.

I often use the following metaphor when I introduce the SST to the person I support through their person care process.

Imagine you have bought a ticket for a theatre performance. You walk in the theatre, take your seat and wait for the play to begin. After some forty minutes the curtains are still down and no sign of the actors. You begin feeling a bit nervous. Twenty minutes later you hear voices and noises coming from the stage but the curtains are still down. You start wondering what is going on. Twenty minutes later the curtains are still down. You may begin arguing with the person sitting next to you, you may start shouting in protest, you may pick a fight with somebody, or you may stay seated in your chair thinking about it or writing about it. You may blame yourself for being there, or for being faulty or stupid, because you don't understand what's going on.

You may also think that you are the only one who understands what is happening: you may believe that it is a new alternative form of theatre you are viewing, one which asks the public to imagine what's happening behind the curtains and make their own representations in their minds about how life is on the other side. After all, you do hear noises and voices coming from there, don't you?

Well, whether you like it or not. This is a metaphor of your life. You get here, take your place and would like to enjoy the show. You won't be fully able to do so until you lift the curtains (or somebody else does it for you). The two huge dichotomies-curtains (positive and negative, good and bad, right and wrong) are preventing you from connecting with real life, with what is being performed on the stage. You have a choice: carry out one or more of the behaviours shown in my example or lift the curtains and make a new start.

Once the curtains are up everything is possible. You may decide to sit down, relax and enjoy the show. You may wish to join in the performance in a variety of ways (i.e. as a main actor, an extra, a member of the technical team, a musician, etc.). You may choose to do something this side of the stage (i.e. selling ice cream, assisting disabled persons getting in and out of the theatre, etc.). Once the curtains are up we can see clearly and real life may begin.

The SST upgrade makes a difference in our lives because it frees us from the shackles of the dichotomies: positive and negative, good or bad, right or wrong. It allows us to walk upright, as humans deserve to, in the land of what is Healthy, Useful and Helpful. That's where Leonardo's Bridge has now finally led you.

Activities Box 35.

Time for your *PAL* …
Think about the SST. Have you ever closed your day in the past? If you have, how did you go about it and what differences do you find in the SST way of doing it?

and for your *BIT.*
Start practising the SST on a daily basis.

Chapter 10

Dimensions & Perspectives

"No matter how difficult the past, you can always begin again today."

Buddha (1)

Thirteenth step
The intrapersonal dimension and your past

Practising the first thirteen steps of this person care programme will have helped distance yourself from unhealthy habits, negative feelings and rational concerns. However, one of the core messages of IPC is that learning is a life long process and learning to take care of yourself is no exception. We learn through experience and we experience through learning and, in so doing, we enrich ourselves personally and professionally as time goes by.

Now that you are in a safer place, you don't want to go back to where you were before. The three steps that make up this chapter will show you how to stay in this healthy, useful and helpful country for as long as you wish. However, before we see what you are required to do to gain citizenship of this wonderful land, let me clarify one important point. When do you know that you have left behind your troubles for good and you are never going to relapse again?

I have worked with persons that had been binge drinking (i.e. fifteen pints of beer in one night three times a week, or one bottle of wine every night for months) or chain-smoking (i.e. 60 cigarettes a day for years) or vomiting (i.e. making themselves sick not less than three times a day for years). In such cases, when do you think we can say that these persons have reached the safe land?

If the beer drinker would start drinking two pints a night twice a week and kept it like that for six months, would you consider them arrived at the other side of Leonardo's Bridge? I would. If the wine drinker would begin drinking one glass of wine with their supper and kept it like that for five months, would you consider them arrived? I would.

If the chain-smoker would stop smoking, and kept it like that for a year, would you consider them arrived? I would. If the bulimic would stop vomiting and kept it like that for eight months, would you consider them arrived? I surely would.

So, what happens if the beer drinker partakes in a stag night, gets drunk and drinks ten pints of beer? What if the wine drinker celebrates their team victory in the premiership and drinks two bottle of wine in one night? What if the smoker goes to a conference and lights up a cigarette before and after their speech? What if the bulimic changes house and job in a matter of weeks and makes themselves sick twice in a week? Would I consider these persons back to square one again? Of course, not.

We are humans. We are not computers. The simple fact that we may have an occasional relapse of an old unhealthy habit does not mean that we have gone back to be that old person again. We do know that relapses tend to decrease in frequency and severity with time, because we learn through experience how to prevent, defuse and manage potential triggers.

Even if some persons take a bit longer to consolidate their new healthy habits, would you say that binge drinking every six months is the same thing as doing it three times a week? Would you say that getting drunk every time your team wins a premiership title is the same thing as drinking every night? Would you say that smoking two cigarettes in a year is the same as smoking 60 a day? Would you say that vomiting twice a week every eight months is the same thing as doing it every day for years?

The point is: we are too hard on ourselves and we take life too seriously. The answer is: take it easy and don't be afraid of getting to know who you are. The more you know about how you function and respond to different situations, the more relaxed you will be about your life's choices and events. So, who are you?

Well, before I show you how to travel within yourself to discover who you really are, I think it would be useful to first take a closer look at what kind of society we live in. This will help us appreciate the powerful forces we interact with as we go about our daily vicissitudes.

The interaction between ourselves and our environment originates our personal conditions (i.e. happiness or sadness). Our capacity for dealing with the above interaction is strongly impaired by what I would define as '*the disguising factor*'.

The disguising factor represents the basic fact that the consumer society, by marketing resources as needs, in its pursuit of increasing the occasions and opportunities for our spending capacity, reduces us to a confused state, which may easily trigger unhealthy behaviours.

Let us take food, as a first example. The primary importance of food is its nutritional value. The secondary aspects of food are: its taste, its look and the rapidity with which you can eat it. Consumer society wants us to eat more than our body would ever need – in terms of nutritional requirements – so it bombards us with adverts that emphasise all the secondary appealing aspects of food. The result: we are eating too many saturated fats, sugars and processed stuff, thus creating the conditions for our poor physical health.

Let us take sex, now, as another example. The primary importance of sex for some is its procreative end. Others view sex primarily as a way of joyfully sharing an experience of love with somebody who is really special to them. The secondary aspects are: the amount of pleasure we take in it, the number of times we have it, the number of partners we sleep with and their looks. Consumer society wants us to invest heavily in our looks, so it bombards us with adverts which emphasise all the secondary aspects of sex. The result: we are too concerned about the external, artificial appearance of our partners depriving ourselves of the much needed real affection coming from meaningful relationships, thus creating the conditions for our poor psychological health.

Either way, consumer society treats us like idiots, who are 'valued' for their spending power rather than for their intellectual, emotional or spiritual faculties.

Consumer society's motto is: "shop until you drop."

Integrated Person Care's motto is: "care until you share."

The role of the parent has always been a difficult one to perform, throughout all ages of human civilisation. However, as a result of the powerful impact of the disguising factor on our lives, parents nowadays are faced with even more challenges.

They may, therefore, unwittingly sow the seeds of insecurity in their offspring by enormously spoiling them from a very early age. This very often results in their sons and daughters' inability to connect with real life in later adolescence and young adulthood.

When parents do everything for them or place them on a high pedestal, their children develop either the perceptual process of overestimating the risk in a situation and underestimating their personal resources for dealing with it (i.e. failing to turn up for university examinations, feeling addicted to unhealthy behaviours), or the opposite process of underestimating the risk and overestimating their resource for coping (getting too easily into debt, binge drinking on a regular basis). Either way what is missing is the balance coming from first hand life experiences in childhood and early adolescence.

Now, I am not saying this because I am blaming a persons' lack of self-esteem on bad parenting and attributing to this the cause our unhealthy behaviours later in life. I have dedicated my previous book to all parents, paying tribute to the difficulty of their role. To the contrary, I am observing this to bring you the good news that it is never too late to learn and change. Truth is, human behaviours do not simplistically follow the physical law of cause and effect and each behaviour may originate from a complex mix of internal and external factors.

That's where getting to know who you are comes in. By acquiring a clear awareness of your present strengths and weaknesses, you will be in a position to consolidate the former and work on the latter, thus ensuring that your life experience becomes a healthy, peaceful and satisfying one.

Before we see how you can become fully aware of who you are, there is just one point I would like to clarify. Some people believe, either spontaneously or as a result of being brainwashed through years of psychoanalysis, that the past is past and you cannot change it.

Therefore, if you were unlucky with your parenting and early childhood experiences you are cursed for the rest of your life and will carry this heavy heap of rubbish with you wherever you go. The best you could hope for, to stay with this view, would be to gain a better understanding of the sort of garbage you are carrying around. This is supposed to help you bear the weight and ease the pain.

Stop this nonsense. NOW! Free yourself from the paws of therapists who make a living out of helping you carry your weight around. Free yourself from the iron chains and leaden balls they have tied to your ankle.

Naturally, we are not able to jump in a time-machine, go back to our past and change it: this is not what I mean.

My point is: our past and our experience of it changes as we grow and change. When we are stuck where we are, nothing changes, including our past. When we grow and learn and develop, our past changes with us, because the way we relate to it and experience it has also changed.

As kids, our family table, the one where we used to have lunch and supper all together, might have looked huge, as adults it seems of a normal size, if not smallish. Why is that? The table is still the same. Yes, exactly! The table is still the same but two important things have changed: we have physically grown up and, as a result, we have now a different appreciation of its size and we have visited many more houses and places and we have seen much bigger tables.

No matter what has happened in our past, we are humans, we can change. We can, first, distance ourselves from it and, then, learn how to perceive it in a completely different light. Remember: we learn through experience and we experience through learning.

This is how, in my view, we deal with traumas. Talking about traumatic events (i.e. basic debriefing) or asking persons to relive them (catharsis, so dear to Freud) in the hope of eliciting some sort of release, has proved to be of no benefit whatsoever and, in some cases, even plainly detrimental.

To help sufferers of traumatic events, some practitioners have achieved good results by using Eye Movement Disensitization Reprocessing (EMDR), a simple technique where persons are led to focus on basic bodily activities, such as following an item (i.e. the practitioner's finger) with their sight while, at the same time, recollecting their traumatic experience. I have obtained very good results by utilising my step-by-step person care approach: traumatised persons felt significantly better than before.

Life can bring us sorrow. Life can bring us understanding, peace of mind and joy. Life is not a persecutor or a rescuer. Life is life, that's all. The sooner we become aware of it the better.

So, stop moaning and blaming your current problems on your father, your mother, your siblings, your school or the weather of the place where you grew up (too cloudy or too sunny, too cold or too hot).

Start taking responsibility for your life. Make a new start. Begin a new journey of exploration within and around you. Now!

First of all, create some time for yourself (a few slots of at least one hour each during the next few days, better if not on consecutive days) and follow the steps below. Begin your self-exploration activities each time with the BBR, the IB and the 3Bs. Each time, close your activities with the 3Bs or the 3Bs + the PA.

1. On the first day, write down a list made of ten 'I am…' statements (i.e. 'I am a good listener', 'I am a lousy dancer'). Jot them down without over-analysing them. Go with the flow. Write the first things coming up and do not change the statements once you have written them down. Place this list in a folder somewhere safe.

2. On the second day, write a second 'I am…' list, without looking at the first list. Then, write down another list made of a minimum of ten things that you value in yourself.

3. On the third day, write a third 'I am…' list, without looking at the previous ones. Then, write down another list made of the things that you see as your weaknesses.

4. On the fourth day, write a fourth 'I am…' list, without looking at the previous ones. Then, write down another list made of the things that you like about your current situation.

5. On the fifth day, write a fifth 'I am…' list, without looking at the previous ones. Then, write down another list made of the things that you dislike about your current situation.

6. On the sixth day, write a sixth 'I am…' list, without looking at the previous ones. Then, write down another list made of the things that make you happy and that you would very much like to keep because they are part of the way you feel, think and behave towards yourself and to others.

7. On the seventh day, write a seventh 'I am…' list, without looking at the previous ones. Then, write down another list made of the things that don't make you happy and that you would very much like to change in the way you feel, think and behave towards yourself and to others.

8. On the eighth day, you calmly read aloud the seven 'I am…' lists. Then, reflect on what you have written and if you notice any meaningful changes from the first lists to the last ones. Finally, make a list of the things you believe in.

9. On the ninth day, you calmly read aloud all the other lists. Then, reflect on what you have written. What do they say about you? Finally, make a list of the things you find interesting.

One story, many lives.

I think it could be useful to offer now a letter written to me by a lady I had seen a couple of years ago. I have called this section 'one story, many lives' because I am sure many of you will identify themselves, partially or totally, with her experience.

My Story

I began my search almost 15 years ago, maybe longer now. I had no idea at the time that my search would lead me to a consulting room in central London at the beginning of February 2002.

One of the first questions I was asked was: "What do you want out of this?" It only took me a small moment to reply: "Peace".

I had become a non-person. I was numb and disconnected from life and living. I had grown up with many responsibilities. I had become dedicated to everyone else's needs and concerns. I was always on my best behaviour and did everything I was told. The last thing I wanted was to cause more dis-ease in our lives. Of course these responsibilities were placed on me by myself. I discovered later, that they gave me purpose and made me feel needed and valued.

So I became a little adult at the age of 7 or so. Everything I did or touched I had to succeed at. I gave everything my best by challenging and disciplining my 'self' all of the time. I was very hard on my 'self' yet very empathic and forgiving of others. I was never good enough, never strong enough, too female, too weak, not intelligent enough and unsatisfactory.

These words became my mantra. They became my focus, my drive. They encouraged me to go harder, faster, deeper. I lived by their energy and their energy alone. I imagined I was a racehorse, training for racing perfection.

It is amazing how I had nurtured these thoughts to punish myself and it was never enough. I had managed to turn all of my external chaos inwardly and blame myself. I was condemned.

The more power I gave to my mantra the more I was becoming disconnected from my family, my friends, my dreams, my passions and me. This focus at the beginning had protected me and cocooned me. It had kept me busy accomplishing.

I was always away from the house, at school, at ballet, at competitive swimming, at gymnastics and part time jobs. I kept time racing, so I wouldn't have to stop and think. I was constantly on the move never resting in one place for long. I was wearing a life jacket, but not just for emergencies, I was wearing it permanently.

My life jacket was a protective barrier from the world, it wasn't saving me, my life jacket was drowning me.

Before I knew it I was lost. I knew no other way. The accomplishments had become constant punishments. The achievements were never satisfactory. The rewards were empty and people's compliments were hollow. I heard nothing and tasted nothing. I was dead.

My 'unlearning' was the most difficult exercise I ever undertook, but because of that fact I took it up as my new challenge. I gave it one thousand percent, dedicating all my energies to it. The reality of having to sit down and be honest to another human being was petrifying. I was thrown from being totally committed to the project to wanting to completely abandon it. I was in, and then I was out. I was tuned in, and then turned off.

My energies had to be re-trained and re-focused. They were not ready for the new territory in which they needed to belong in order for me to survive. My feelings were threatened; they were comfortable where they were. They were content and understood their domain. I had to build them a new house and they did not want to move in. They were quite comfortable living the way they were.

My entire world was being viewed from another window of the same house. Essentially I had to learn to trust that good would come to me, that I was not being punished and that my life was a worthy one. I had to take a step forward. The first thing I remember that made me listen was a simple question, which I asked myself: "Do you want to live or do you want to die?" "If you continue this way we will find you dead lying by the toilet." This was my trigger. It shot through my numbness and jolted me awake.

The truth I have learned is painful. I have learned that life is hard. I have learned that to live is to feel. I have learned to cry and to laugh, to be sad and to feel joy. I realised that I had long been dead but now I am alive. I feel.

I would encourage everyone to take a risk and discover the hidden parts of you that you have long trained into submission. They are part of you. They need to be cherished and understood. You cannot escape them. They have unbounded wisdom and will find a way to show themselves eventually. In order to be at peace, I needed to listen to all of me.

My life has become rich. I have become a lover, a sister, an aunty, and a daughter. I am learning new things every day. At the beginning my voices were like thunder in my head. Sometimes the rain clouds break again, pouring all over me, but somehow they don't wet me like they used to. I now treasure these opportunities to continue my growth.

Now, I can say: "I am at peace".

Activities Box 36.

Time for your *PAL* …
Carry out the self-exploration activities above.

and for your *BIT*.
Discuss the outcome of your self-exploration activities with your travel mate.

Dimensions & Perspectives

Fourteenth step
The personal dimension and your present

Now that you know yourself a bit better, it is time to put this knowledge to good use and see how you can improve the quality of your personal life. As a start let's consider how the social environment we live in impacts on the personal choices we make by introducing what I would define as '*the speed factor*'.

As the German sociologist Bernd Guggenberger notes:
   "We live as forgetful beings under the spell of speed, we carry on as if we were always travelling and bringing with us the absolute minimum required in terms of tradition, affection and personal identity. We have become 'chameleons of ethics' leaving behind great passions and high ideals because they were the cause of difficulties and pathos. In the celebration of the 'here and now', feelings, like fashion, are quickly born and rapidly fade away. Qualities are not to be really possessed, but effectively shown: there is no time to discover and evaluate them, that would require a long relationship, so we relate to others merely on the basis of how they appear to be." (2)

Bellino also observes how:
   "The overwhelming rapidity of social change (Goethe's 'Das Veloziferische') has originated not only the crisis of ideologies, but the crisis of our personal planning capacity, too."(3)

Incredibly high rhythms of personal life within a rapidly changing social environment inevitably take their toll on our physical and psychological well-being. Our species has become what it is as a result of millions of years of evolution and it has had no time to catch up with what has happened in the past 150 years – that is, an insignificantly short time, in evolutionary terms.

Try to imagine how our life was in 1856. How many sources of stress and anxiety can you think of? Can you hear your office telephones ringing, or the trill originated by the mobile phone in your pocket?

Can you hear the noise coming from busy streets and the roar of car engines while you are waiting at the bus stop? Can you enjoy healthy breathing within a packed underground train or the comforting view of the evening news flooding your auditory channels with information whose quality is finely matched by the stuff they are making us eat and bravely call 'food'?

The past 150 years have severely put us to the test, and the speed factor, with its deep and far-reaching implications for our physical and psychological health, has been largely underestimated by mainstream psychotherapy, which has mostly been concerned with relieving some of its effects (i.e. stress, anxiety) rather than with confronting their sources.

The stress you suffer as a result of the sheer speed at which you live is often made worse by the tendency of companies towards downsizing their job force. Losing a job is not just stressful for who actually loses it. Those who are left behind feel the added pressure of knowing that they have been spared this time around and often work more as fewer employees now deal with the same workload. Those still employed bear also the extra worry that there could be more layoffs in the future, which is even worst, psychologically, than knowing for sure that they will indeed lose their job in a given time in the future.

In such circumstances, it is not uncommon that persons are drawn towards extreme personal and professional choices, like leaving everything behind and escaping somewhere else – often as a consequence of a nervous break down – or throwing themselves even more into their professional activities, thus leaving virtually no room for their personal life. Coming up with balanced practical alternatives becomes naturally difficult in these situations. However, embracing the challenge of making our life a better place within our present environment represents, in almost all cases, the sensible way forward.

Here is a step-by-step indication of how you can go about your personal orientation activity:

1. First, choose somebody you trust and whose opinion you value. In the end, you will be the one to decide how to go about your personal issues, but it does help to have somebody to talk to. Sometimes good ideas come up as a result of interacting with the appropriate person.

2. Then, start looking after your body by:

a) Making a little time for yourself every day (i.e. leisure time, friends and family).

b) Slowing down the pace of your daily activities. Practising regularly the BBR will help you do this.

c) Begin exercising nicely and gently every day (even room exercises will do).

3. Next, nurture your emotional self by connecting with each moment of your day. Live fully every little thing that you do. Practising the IB and the 3Bs can help you do this.

4. Finally, give a boost to your rational self by living as a 'special' person. The exercises carried out during the previous step, where you gave yourself the opportunity to know more about who you are, can be put to use now. Special persons live a special life, one that is full of special things. You know what you like and what makes you happy, so go for it!

Another important issue worth addressing here is the close association between the personal choices you make and how happy you are with your professional life. I have worked with many persons whose personal life was pretty ok, but whose dissatisfaction with their job brought about considerable suffering and often triggered unhealthy behaviours (i.e. vomiting, drinking) or unwanted conditions (i.e. loss of sleep, bad temper). As a matter of fact, the more we become aware of our potential (in emotional as well as professional terms), the more we suffer as a result of the gap we perceive between it and our current personal or professional situation.

If this is happening to you, I would advise creating some time to re-think your career and think about your professional orientation. To help you do that, you may follow the step-by-step guidance offered below. The goal of the following activity is to come up with a grid whose fully completed version will provide you with a clear indication of your career aspiration.

I strongly recommend you to carry out this activity, step-by-step, exactly as it is indicated. This is because even the slightest tendency towards jumping to conclusions and predicting the outcome of the next step would compromise the usefulness of this exercise.

Please note that two sample professional orientation grids are provided in Appendix D and E. The first is blank, the second is fully completed and scored.

This is how to complete your **professional orientation** grid:

1. Make some time for yourself during the next few days. Allow, at least, one hour at a time and a couple of days in between each session.

2. Carry out a brain-storming activity where you write down your favourite areas of interest (i.e. music, health, economy, tourism). A feasibility assessment (i.e. would I be able to make a living working in this field?) is neither required nor appropriate, at this stage.

3. Identify professional roles of interest within each of the areas above. For example, for music it could be a journalist specialising in jazz, disc jockey, band manager or event organiser; for health it could be a nurse or counsellor; for economy it could be an analyst or trader; for tourism could be holiday representative, travel agent or guide.

4. Allow a 3-4 day break and, without looking at the above list of professional roles, write down a list of characteristics that you would value in your professional life (i.e. opportunity to develop personally, working environment, making a difference in people's life, financial reward, etc.).

5. Carry out an assessment of the importance of the above characteristics when compared to each other. For example, you may attribute a normal value to some (i.e. working environment and financial reward), and more value to others (i.e. personal development and making a difference in people's life). Once you have created your scale of values, give a weight to each value (i.e. working environment = normal value = weight 1; personal development = double value = weight 2; making a difference in people's lives = triple value = weight 3).

6. Enter your roles and characteristics in your grid, as showed in Appendix D. Do not enter the weight of each characteristic in their cell, as you want to make sure that your initial scores are not affected by the concomitant appraisal of a characteristic's weight.

7. Make as many copies of the grid as the professional roles you have identified and, on different days, score just one role on each sheet by entering your value in the Initial Score (IC) cells. This is done to ensure that you don't look at previous values as you score subsequent roles. I would recommend the use of a 1 to 10 scale for your scoring.

8. Transfer your scores on one sheet, as in Appendix E. Calculate their weighted values and, then add them up. The results will show you which roles would best match your desired characteristics.

9. Now, it's time to carry out a feasibility assessment. Starting from the role with the highest score, assess how feasible it is for you to train or re-train in the chosen roles. You may also wish to allow for a transitional period where you carry on your present occupation and train part-time for the new. You may then resign from the current job as soon as you feel ready to go for the new one. Some have also opted for working part-time in the old position, to make sure that enough money was coming in to pay for the bills, and began practising part-time the new activity. Some have actually found that they were already in the right job and carrying out this exercise provided them with a renewed motivation to continue and with a clearer insight into their personal issues (i.e. difficult relationships or unhealthy habits).

I have gone through the above process with a number of persons over the past four years. In the end, they were surprised at how such a simple step-by-step activity enabled them to turn bleak scenarios, where apparently no way out could be found, into workable and stimulating alternatives.

Activities Box 37.

Time for your *PAL* …
Think about the pace of life just 150 years ago. Then think about its speed now. What similarities and differences do you find?

and for your *BIT.*
Practise the above 4-step personal orientation activity.

Fifteenth step
The interpersonal dimension and your future

When we experience personal distress we are likely to withdraw from social contacts. Rationally we know that this is not appropriate and that isolating ourselves from the world does not do us any favour, but when you are there in the middle of the emotional storm picking up radio signals from the control room becomes very difficult.

Taking some time off to give ourselves the occasion to reflect on past events, current choices and future goals, is absolutely fine. There is a value in sadness and it lies in the chance that it allows us to reassess our decisions and readjust our route in the light of difficult times and situations, thus providing us with the opportunity to add meaning to our life, in spite of ever-changing external circumstances.

The art of balancing the primordial survival instinct of looking after ourselves with the equally primeval drive towards interacting satisfactorily with fellow human beings will be the topic of this step. You will learn here how to improve your interpersonal relationships and how to deal with difficult ones.

First, I would like you to be fully aware that persons are not just what they are, as physical entities. To us, each person we meet also represents the metaphor for something or someone else. So, for example, when a fifty-three year old man leaves behind a long-term relationship to start a fling with a much younger woman, what the man sees in her is not just youth or possibly beauty, but his own lost youth and his own lost beauty and in embracing this adventure he is trying to recapture them.

What's wrong with this? You may ask. Well, living as members of a community does not attract only a number of legal and civic duties (i.e. paying your taxes or disposing sensibly of your domestic waste). It also involves adherence to an interpersonal moral code whereby persons abide by a behavioural and communicative style informed by decency and honesty.

Therefore, if a single man has chosen to go from one fling to another and he has made this clear to the women he dates, from a psychological point of view I don't see anything unhealthy in this. But, when a man (often married or already committed to a long-term relationship) deals with women like they were toys to play with, performs deceptively the role of the adoring boyfriend for as long as he has his fun and then throws them away when he has become bored with them, this person is sowing with full hands the seeds of personal distress causing misery to a number of fellow human beings.

Naturally, I can also offer a number of healthy examples. Like the case of the man who decides to befriend an elderly couple because his parents died when he was still young, or the lady who chose to adopt a Romanian boy after her own son died in a car accident. Humans have the capacity to spread healthy seeds and harvest, as a result, plenty of consolation and joy.

Now, let's take a closer look at interpersonal interactions: what are their main ingredients?

We do know that they are about sharing, but what is it that we are sharing with someone else at a given moment of our life?

There are two fundamental components to each relationship, whether we are in the presence of a personal interaction (i.e. siblings, friends, girlfriends) or a professional one (i.e. school mates, work colleagues). These components are intimacy and togetherness.

Intimacy consists of the meaningful situations we share, like open dialogues and confidences, physical closeness, sexual intercourse and other significant experiences. Intimacy is about giving and receiving. It may have its ups and downs like the tidal waves. One day you give, another you receive. You just go with the flow and enjoy it.

Togetherness consists of the motivation and willingness to share our interests and life projects. Please note that we say 'share' and not 'unconditionally accept' or 'abide by', because you can, for example, share somebody's interest in the arts without feeling obliged spending hours in art galleries every time you visit a new town, or share your colleague's enthusiasm for a new project without totally agreeing with him on how to develop it. Togetherness is about team work and being in the same boat rowing in the same direction. Togetherness is about mutual support.

Healthy relationships are the ones where there are elements of both components. When relationships are made only of elements of just one component, they are unbalanced and sooner or later problems will arise. Humans are not perfect and perfect relationships are not of this world. That's why it is so important to appreciate two main points:

a) Work is always in progress: if you want to make the most of an interpersonal interaction, be prepared to work on it, nicely, gently and, above all, constantly.

b) It takes two to tango: one thing is having ups and downs, as part of the normal games of intimacy, another is having a major unbalance at the togetherness level.

So, how do we work practically on improving our interpersonal skills?

Lesson 1. Relating is an art.

Relating at the interpersonal level is an art, like relating at the intrapersonal and personal ones, not an exact science. Relating is the art of integrating intimacy and togetherness. You learn through experience and you experience through learning. So, to make sure that you are able to practise this art proficiently and satisfactorily you want to learn how to create a balance.

An interpersonal balance is made up of five elements: both persons have the time and the space for being on their own, both persons have the time and the space for being with others, there is enough time and space for sharing intimacy and togetherness. If one of the above elements is missing, a relationship, of any nature, will not go very far.

Lesson 2. Creating an internal balance.

Healthy relationships comprise two balanced persons. If one isn't, the interpersonal interaction will not work. So, first of all, make sure that you are aware of where you are, at a given moment in time. Are you happy with your physical condition? Are you at peace with yourself? Do you think you are connected with your rational resources? If the answers to the above questions are not completely affirmative, do your own work first.

I once saw a pleasant lady who came to me because of difficulties in the relationship with her new partner.

She felt very close to him, there were many things she liked about him and she was sure that he felt the same about her, but they seemed to have problems in communicating with each other, which would often result in unnecessary arguing and this started exacting its toll by making their interactions increasingly difficult.

She was genuinely puzzled when I suggested to work first on her own internal balance, as she was expecting me to address interpersonal issues straightaway. However, she took my word for it. After four meetings and before we even got started on their communication styles, she told me that her partner's behaviour had changed so significantly and their relating improved so much that it was not necessary to get into the second stage of our programme.

How come? Simply put, persons respond to how we are, even before they process how we relate to them. Working on her internal balance made her realise that psychologically she was not in a comfortable place and that this uneasiness was filtering through to her partner who misinterpreted it as a sign that there was something wrong with him and their relationship, whereas her issues were of a different – and internal – nature.

By improving her internal balance she started sending out different signals (i.e. more relaxed and peaceful behaviours) to her partner, who, responded accordingly.

They say you cannot change the world. Well, I don't know about that. All I know is that when I am surrounded by nervous (or stressed, tired, etc.) persons this may affect me. Likewise I do feel different when in the company of relaxed (or happy, easy-going, etc.) persons.

When we work on our internal balance we become the persons we would like to be with, spreading healthy vibes all around and impacting in a helpful way on each person we meet.

If you feel balanced, you may wish to understand if your interlocutor is balanced too. If it is clear that they are not, see what you can do to help them. As we have just seen, being consistently balanced yourself can already help.

You don't want to impose your own person care model onto them (i.e. 'here, read this book and sort yourself out'), but you may ask how they are and if they know how to take care of their issues. Not knowing what to do or how to go about it is not a crime.

The point is, you don't want to waste your time with somebody who is not willing to look after themselves (because they don't want to or because they are not ready as yet).

Lesson 3. Creating an external balance.

If you notice a genuine interest in the person you are relating to in working on themselves and in improving your relationship there are a few things you can do:

- ➢ Make time to openly talk about your relationship.

- ➢ See if you can find a common ground to use as a safe base to leave from and come back to during your conversations.

- ➢ Be aware of your own behaviour and be ready to accept the other person's feedback on it (i.e. at times we are not aware of the tone of our voice, the expression of our face or the posture we assume, which can unwittingly become abusive or threatening).

- ➢ Agree on 'response delay' behaviours to adopt when one of the two doesn't feel ready to engage in a conversation about the relationship. So, for example, you may agree that it is ok to move to another room for a few minutes, or to colour code some behaviours and make the other aware of their colour at that moment in time ('oh dear, you are becoming deep purple love…'), or to write notes about what is bothering you which are then placed in a box, a pot or a drawer that the other can go and read when they feel ready.

As you can see, the above practical suggestions can be easily applied both in personal interactions (i.e. a sibling or a partner), and in professional ones (i.e. a work colleague or a fellow student).

Lesson 4. Learning to let go.

There is a time to work on a relationship and there is a time to let it go. Interpersonal interactions are supposed to be a 50-50 endeavour.

Sometimes the balance can go 60-40 or even 70-30 or 80-20, and that's fine provided that we go back to a point where both persons do their bit by rowing in the same direction.

However, many are stuck in co-dependent relationships, where they end up taking a lot of abuse and grief as a result of having become addicted either to another person, or to what this person represents to them (remember, persons are also metaphors for something or someone else).

The point is: what is unhealthy for you cannot be healthy for someone else. I will clarify this with a real life example.

A young woman came to me complaining about her relationship with her partner. He was a heroine addict and had been feeding his addiction first with his own resources and then with hers.

After years of empty promises of the kind 'I will clean myself up as from tomorrow, next week or the beginning of the month', she had had enough but she felt unable to leave him when he seemed to need her most.

As you can see, she was playing the rescuer. For a number of reasons that it would not be appropriate to mention here, she had been performing the rescuer, the caring person who was always there ready to offer everything she had.

She did not realise how, in doing that, she was keeping her partner in a victim condition, thus reinforcing a situation that was deeply unhealthy for both.

When we take full responsibility for somebody's life, we take away from them the precious opportunity to learn how to take care of themselves.

When she finally decided to give him an ultimatum ("either you commit yourself to a rehabilitation programme or I'll leave and start a new life without you", he replied, at first, despondently ("go, I'll find somebody else").

Now, he was given back the choice to do what he wanted to do with his life. She left and made a new start, which brought her a new job and a fulfilling relationship.

A few weeks later he decided to clean himself up for good and about a year later he wrote a wonderful letter to her. He thanked her for having made him realise how deep down he had got into his addiction and acknowledged how, by dissociating herself from this deeply hurtful experience, she gave him the chance to look and see how he was wasting his life. He was now back at work again and in a new relationship.

If you are currently stuck in a co-dependent relationship or you know somebody in such a situation, what you can do is to make the most of the few moments of clarity that you or your friend will still have and either go through this person care programme from the beginning or seek professional help. Remember: if you partner is not willing to change, making a new start will benefit both of you. So, if you really care about somebody, sometimes letting go of them could be the most appropriate thing to do.

Lesson 5. Getting out of the unhealthy triangle.

As we have seen above, we may find ourselves trapped in an unhealthy and self-perpetuating victim-persecutor-rescuer spiral. When this happens, now you know what to do – and how to go – about it. To help you get straight to the point, I have provided an index of the exercises introduced in this guide in Appendix E.

To briefly sum up, if you feel you are in the 'victim' situation, practise the BBR, the Language Point and the SST. This will help you get out of the triangle, rather than moving to the 'persecutor' situation.

If you feel you are playing the 'persecutor', practise the BBR, the IB, the 3Bs, the PA and the SST. This will help you out of the triangle, rather than moving to the 'rescuer' situation.

If you feel you are acting as the 'rescuer', practise the BBR, the 3As and the SST. This will help you out of the triangle, rather than moving back to the 'victim' situation.

Naturally, the above suggestions are only meant as a shortcut to help you out in 'emergency' functioning. You are warmly encouraged to follow through the whole person care programme from the start, in the appropriate order.

Activities Box 38.

Time for your *PAL* …
Think about one personal and one professional relationship you are currently engaged in. How balanced do you think they are, both internally and externally?

and for your *BIT.*
Practise the above lessons.

Chapter 11

Notes for the journey ahead

"The only thing necessary for the triumph of evil
is for good men to do nothing."

Edmund Burke (1)

"It is man who makes truth great,
not truth which makes man great."

Confucius

The 21st century Renaissance.

The Integrated Person Care programme is part of a wider cultural framework which I have called 'the 21st century Renaissance'.

The 15th century Renaissance consisted of a revival in arts and literature which originated in Florence: its main aspiration consisted of a rediscovery of the human being and of the natural world.

After centuries of bowing to external and intangible forces, human beings were finally seen as their own masters and educators.

People and environments were represented as they really were, rather than as they should be: pure geniuses like Brunelleschi, Masaccio and Donatello paved the way for the extraordinary accomplishments of Raffaello and Leonardo da Vinci.

The 21st century Renaissance encourages all of us to create the conditions for a reawakening of our connection both with the healing power of the life forces **within** us – the 'biological' (i.e. breathing and energy) as well as the 'creative' ones (i.e. arts and music) – and **around** us (the natural world and fellow human beings).

It also invites us to open up our hearts and share this awareness with each other.

Our message for you is:

"Join the 21st century Renaissance. Start giving in to your spontaneity and creativity. Begin taking care of yourself. Now!"

Getting in touch.

Our school offers one-to-one consultations, classes and workshops in IPC and Peaceflow, on a weekly or intensive basis, both in London and abroad (currently in Tuscany).

We also offer one-to-one (or one-to-two) training for health care practitioners in Integrated Person Care and Peaceflow, both in London and abroad. For more information, please get in touch with us at the address below.

I would really appreciate your comments on this little guide. Your feedback and criticism can contribute to helping other sufferers, carers or practitioners. I will use them both in my professional practice and in my next publications. Please forward your opinions to:

Tommaso Palumbo
School of Integrated Person Care
26 Eccleston Street
London
SW1W 9PY
Telephone: 0044 020 7881 0601
Emails: info@personcare.org ~ info@peaceflow.org
Websites: http://www.personcare.org ~ http://www.peaceflow.org

Appendix A

Frequently Asked Questions.

What do I think of diets?

Diets are never the solution to your issues and are often the cause of your problems. Many develop serious illnesses and eating disorders as a result of a diet. So, what shall we do? You want to take care of your body by applying the advice and suggestions offered in this guide. There's no need to embark on yet another diet.

How much carbohydrates should you eat?

Carbs provide fuel. So how much your body requires depends on how you use it. Bear in mind that up to one third of the energy you produce is used by your brain alone, so whatever you do make sure that you eat a good source of carbs at each meal.

How much proteins should you eat?

You have developed your muscle system and bones structure, thanks to the consumption of proteins. The functioning of the immune system requires proteins too. Naturally, adults still require proteins to keep their muscle tone and bone density and for the production of certain hormones – like the one regulating the functioning of the thyroid. A healthy male should eat between 50 and 55 grams of protein a day. A healthy female between 45 and 50. To give you a practical idea of what that means, consider that when you eat 100 grams of fish or meat you provide your body with approximately 25 grams of proteins.

How much fat should you eat?

State Registered Dieticians say: *"Fat is often given a bad name. We only need to watch the television advertisements or walk around the supermarket to be reminded that we should be reducing the level of fat in our diet. This is often taken to extremes. Fat is **essential** for life. It is recommended that between 30 and 35% of our energy intake **should** come from fat. There are three types of fat – saturated fats, polyunsaturated fats and monounsaturated fats. **We need all types of fat in our diet.** No fat is 'bad'.*

*Following a diet **too low in fat** is likely to:*

1. *Lead to a greater preoccupation with food. This could increase a persons risk of bingeing.*
2. *Make you feel hungry. Fat helps increase satiety levels. Including fat at mealtimes reduces the likelihood of snacking between meals.*
3. *Lead to nutritional deficiencies.*

For females, approximately 20 to 25% of the body weight should be fat. For males it is approximately 10 to 15%. Levels lower than this are likely to lower resistance to disease, cause weakness, irritability and effect fertility.

*Fat is **essential** to:*

- *Keep us warm.*
- *Protect our internal organs from impacts such as a fall.*
- *Provide us with essential fatty acids, which we need to eat on a **daily** basis. These are essential for brain function and in the prevention of heart disease. Essential fatty acids are extremely important to the growing foetus for normal brain development.*
- *Contribute to the structure of blood vessels.*
- *Coat our skin with a thin but essential layer. Detergents remove this layer causing dry skin. The skin will secrete more fats which build up to normal levels after a few days.*
- *Transport cholesterol around the body. Cholesterol levels are often raised if you are avoiding fat. The exact explanation for this is unknown although if you reintroduce more fat into your diet following a period of restriction, your cholesterol level will fall.*
- *Contribute to the structure of hormones, for example oestrogen. For women, reduced oestrogen will have a knock on effect, i.e. lack of periods increasing the risk of osteoporosis.*
- *Provide us with fat soluble vitamins, i.e. vitamin A. This vitamin is required for growth and repair of tissues, i.e. muscles such as your heart". (1)*

Which fats should you favour?

As Meredith Small notes *"...the most dramatic change in what we eat has happened in the past century, with industrialisation and the development of the food industry. Manufacturers favour foods with long shelf lives, so they mostly use soy, corn, palm and cottonseed oil. All contain high amounts of omega-6 fatty acids and very little omega-3, a balance that is further skewed when the oils are hydrogenated to make them keep even longer.*

According to Hibbeln, the average annual consumption of soy oil in the US stands at 11 kilograms, a thousandfold increase in less than 100 years. It accounts for 83 per cent of all the fats we eat. And while we ladle on the omega-6s, most of us eat few of the foods that are high in omega-3s such as oily fish, walnuts, flax seed and olive oil. As a result, our diets now contain 16 times as much omega-6 as omega-3, whereas a century ago we would have been getting about equal amounts of each. 'No body could adjust that fast', says Hibbeln". (2)

Is snacking a healthy or an unhealthy habit?

As Dr Lefever observes: *"Chewing stimulates the appetite centre of the brain. Once stimulated, it remains 'turned on' for about twenty minutes. Grazing between meals can therefore result in a constant feeling of hunger or expectation of food. For the same reason it is possible still to feel hungry after a vast, but rapid, binge." (3)*

Is irregular eating predisposing you to weight gain?

According to the International Journal of Obesity, irregular eating decreases the thermic effect of food compared to regular eating even in thin people, thus the answer is affirmative: irregular eating will predispose to obesity.

How often should you weigh yourselves?

As far as I am concerned, you may as well throw your scale in the bin: scales always tell lies. What is the meaning of a scale value? Does it say anything about how much muscle, bones and fat cells your body is made of? You may be losing weight and be happy by adhering to a very unhealthy diet which is making you lose precious muscle and bone density rather than fat cells. You may be gaining weight thanks to a balanced diet which is making you lose all the unwanted fat zones but is strengthening your muscles and bones. Which option would you choose? Would you rather weigh 55 Kg and be rundown and flabby, or weigh 60 Kg and be fit and slim?

People who go on a diet, are not concerned about numbers! They fret about their shape. They mourn about the loss of not being able to fit in a pair of jeans that they have been able to wear for the past seven years. Now, whether it is realistic to expect that a 25 year old woman may still fit in the same size of trousers she would wear when 18, well that's another issue. The point I am making here is that your scale says nothing about your fitness and shape: it gives you just a meaningless number. Muscle and bones cells are comparatively heavier than fat cells: your scale says nothing about that!

So, what I suggest you to do is to find your 'shape indicator' to help you monitor on a monthly basis how you take care of your body. Choose an item from your wardrobe (i.e. a pair of trousers, a dress, etc) and try it on to check your overall shape and which parts of your body you will like to work on. This way, rather than fretting about a meaningless number, you will be able to focus your energy on specific areas of your body you would like to work on through general or targeted forms of exercise and balanced eating.

How do you know if you are not eating enough?

You will experience any, or a combination, of the following symptoms:

"Emotional
1. Depression
2. Irritability and anxiety
3. Muddled natural instincts
4. Progressive withdrawal and isolation

Behavioural
1. Dramatic increase in preoccupation with food
2. Total devotion to feeding others
3. Eating slowly and chewing thoroughly
4. Increased hunger (intolerable)

Physical
1. Gastro-intestinal discomfort
2. Decreased need for sleep
3. Dizziness, headaches
4. Hypersensitivity to noise and light
5. Reduced strength
6. Hair loss
7. Poor tolerance of cold temperatures" (4)

Are you sugar sensitive?

If you have been brought up eating lots of sugary stuff, chances are that you are. Sugar sensitivity has been linked with alcohol addiction and binge eating. To find out more about this I would warmly recommend the reading of *Potatoes not Prozac*, by Katheleen Des Maisons. The full reference is indicated in the Resources section of this guide.

Are you drinking enough water?

75% of Americans are chronically dehydrated (this finding may apply to half the world's population). In 37% of Americans, the thirst mechanism is so weak that it is often mistaken for hunger. Even mild dehydration will slow down one's metabolism as much as 3%. One glass of water shuts down midnight hunger pangs for almost 100% of the dieters studied in a University of Washington study. Lack of water is the number 1 trigger of daytime fatigue.

Preliminary research indicates that 8-10 glasses of water a day could significantly ease back and joint pain for up to 80% of sufferers. A mere 2% drop in body water can trigger fuzzy short-term memory, trouble with basic math and difficulty focusing on the computer screen or on a printed page. Drinking 5 glasses of water daily decreases the risk of colon cancer by 45%, plus it can slash the risk of breast cancer by 79%, and one is 50% less likely to develop bladder cancer. (5)

Appendix B

General Information About Eating

(reproduced from Dr Robert Lefever's book *'Eating Disorder'*)

Eating should be a pleasure: the taste and process of eating should be enjoyable.

Fluid retention, diabetes, thyroid deficiency and various other medical conditions can have an effect on body weight but can easily be controlled medically and should have no effect on the simultaneous treatment of an eating disorder.

As a general rule for good health one should drink one and a half to two litres (seven to ten cups) of fluid each day.

Bottled sauces are best avoided because many of them contain sugar or white flour or they may be very spicy and stimulate the appetite. They may also blunt the palate so that it becomes progressively less sensitive to delicate flavouring.

Appetite suppressants should be totally avoided because they are addictive. It should be realised that nicotine, caffeine and diet drinks tend to be used as appetite suppressants and these substances are in any case addictive in their own right, whatever the reason for their use.

Laxatives should be avoided because they form part of the binge/purge behavioural addiction component of an eating disorder. Bowel function takes time to return to normal after years of abuse through an eating disorder. Patients with anorexia, for example, will often complain that they are "constipated" when what they mean is that they have the sensation of something in their bowels. This sensation is therefore not due to constipation but to hypersensitivity as a result of years of starvation.

Taking regular exercise is healthy but as little as twenty or thirty minutes a day for three days a week is quite healthy enough. Exercise and the "high" it can produce can become an addiction in itself.

It takes about ten days for the emotional high and subsequent withdrawal symptoms from sugar to clear. Each sugar binge will result in its own withdrawal period.

If you experience any cravings to binge, purge or starve you should share these feelings with someone at the time, if this is possible. Cravings are not something to be ashamed about. Nor are they a sign that things are going badly. Indeed, they are entirely normal and they are common for an addict in early recovery.

So-called "forbidden foods", particularly in anorexic patients, tend to become an obsession. These patients often make lists of forbidden foods – usually fats, meats and carbohydrates – that are all perfectly healthy. This obsession can even sometimes take the form of supposed food allergies and tactical vegetarianism (designed to produce weight loss, rather than from philosophical conviction). When we come into recovery it is important to reconsider what we are prepared to eat.

Meal times should be as regular as possible. Some sufferers find excuses to have breakfast at 5am or put dinner off until 11pm. We need to learn to keep within normal parameters, such as having breakfast at 7-9am, lunch at 12 - 2pm and dinner at 7 - 9pm. These are guidelines only and may not suit shift work. However, it is important to have three meals well spaced throughout the working hours.

Some guidance may be useful on the concept of normal eating, but making out particular "food plans" or having "food sponsors" can be dangerously obsessive. It gives food a power that it does not possess. There is no need to count out exact weights, portions or calories. We need to learn to eat according to genuine physical hunger rather than emotional cravings.

IPC Repertory Grid

IPC Grid		Name:						Date:			
1	Past			Present			Future			**5**	
Similarities	E1	E2	E3	E4	E5	E6	E7	E8	E9	Opposites	
PC1											PC1
PC2											PC2
PC3											PC3
PC4											PC4
PC5											PC5
PC6											PC6
PC7											PC7
PC8											PC8
PC9											PC9
PC10											PC10

203

Appendix D

Professional Orientation Grid (Blank)

	Journalist	Counsellor	Trader	Travel Agent
Working environment				
Financial reward				
Personal development				
Making a difference in people's life				

Appendix E

Professional Orientation Grid (Completed)

	Journalist		Counsellor		Trader		Travel Agent	
	IC	WV	IC	WV	IC	WV	IC	WV
Working environment Weight 1	5	5	6	6	7	7	6	6
Financial reward Weight 1	6	6	5	5	9	9	6	6
Personal development Weight 2	6	12	8	16	5	10	6	12
Making a difference in people's life Weight 3	6	18	8	24	4	12	5	15
		41		51		38		39

Appendix F

Index of Techniques

Technique	Step		Page Number
Magic Box	Third		116
Magic Purse	Third		118
Holy Place	Third		118
K-Technique	Fourth		121
Pre-active Mode	Sixth		132
Basic Body Relaxation (BBR)	Seventh		138
Insight Breathing	Seventh		139
3Bs	Eighth		142
Positive Association (PA)	Ninth		147
Breathing Visualisation Exercise (BVE)	Ninth		149
Language Point	Tenth		154
3As	Eleventh		160
Slide Show Technique	Twelfth		167

Notes

Introduction

See Kornfield (1994), p. 92

1   What is Integrated Person Care?

1. See Kornfield (1994), p. 40

2   Philosophical Concepts

1. Matthew's Gospel, 6:34
2. Kornfield (1994), p. 1
3. De Crescenzo (1983), p. 38
4. Filippani-Ronconi (1994), p. 20
5. Thich Nhat Hanh (1997)
6. De Crescenzo (1986), p. 157
7. Hadot (1999), p. 114
8. Hadot (1999), p. 87
9. Hadot (1999), p. 228
10. Laszlo (1978)
11. Bellino (1988)
12. Furedi (2004), p. 260

3   Psychological Theories

1. See Kornfield (1994), p. 17.
2. Freud (1991), p. 20.
3. Freud (1993).
4. See De Crescenzo (1986), p. 185.
5. Dryden (1999), p. 5.
6. Beck (1991), p. 108.
7. Beck (1991), p. 114.
8. Beck (1991), p. 3.
9. Beck (1991), p. 55.
10. Smail (1993).
11. Lerner and Sheldon (2002), p. 30.
12. Smail (1998), p. 38.
13. Deary (2003).
14. Pinel (2003), p. 66.

15. Northcutt & Kaas (1995) in Pinel (2003).
16. Swanson & Petrovich (1998) in Pinel (2003).
17. Burne (2004).
18. Servan-Schreiber (2004) in Burne (2004).
19. Goleman (1995).
20. Van der Kolk (2002), p. 8.
21. Davidson (2004).Lane & Nadel (2000) in Van der Kolk (2002), p. 12.
22. Farley (2004), p. 42.
23. Farley (2004), p. 42.
24. Farley (2004), p. 42.
25. Servan-Schreiber in Burne (2004).
26. Canter (2002), p. 50.
27. Beck (1991), p. 75.
28. Servan-Schreiber in Burne (2004).
30. Woolf (2001) in Thernstrom (2001).
31. Thernstrom (2001).
32. Rowe (2001), p. 5.
33. Fairburn & Harrison (2003), p. 407.
34. Bettelheim (1982).
35. Bettelheim (1982).
36. Freud (1991).
37. Bettelheim (1982).
38. Jacobs (2002), p. 22.
39. Freud (1933) in Bettelheim (1982).
40. Freud (1933) in Bettelheim (1982).
41. Beck (1991), p. 3.
42. Beck (1991), p. 220.
43. Beck (1991), p. 216
44. Van der Kolk (2002), p. 9.
45. Van der Kolk (2004) in Pointon, p. 11.
46. Lazarus (1997), p. 6.
47. Lazarus (1997), p. 11.
48. Lazarus (1997), p. 31.
49. Lazarus (1997), p. 31.
50. Lazarus (1997), p. 26.
51. Ellis in Dryden (1999), p. 112/p. 117.
52. Lefever (2003), p. 14.

4   Practising PPC

1. Lawrence (1987), p. 33.
2. Burne (2004).
3. Healy (1998) in Palumbo (1999).
4. Canter (2002),   p. 50.
5. Small (2002), p. 34.
6. Lefever (2003), p. 13.
7. Smail (1998), p. 185.
8. Smail (1993).
9. Seligman (2004) in Lawson (2004), p. 34.
10. Lawson (2004).
11. Hirst (2002), p. 23.

5   The Opening Stage

1. Gide in Morelli-Zerbini (1994), p. 34.
2. Bettelheim (1982), p. 55.
3. See Assagioli (1971).

6   Sensations

1. Buddha in Kornfield (1994), p. 5
2. Lefever (2003)

7   Behaviours

1. Buddha in Kornfield (1994), p. 28

8   Emotions

1. Buddha in Kornfield (1994), p. 46
2. Lanza del Vasto (1975)
3. Ippolito in Borrelli & Palumbo (2004), p. 69

9   Thoughts

1. Roshi in Kornfield (1994), p. 29
2. Malley-Morrison (2004)
3. Morelli (2006)
4. Morelli (2006)

Goleman, D. (1995) *Emotional Intelligence*, Glasgow: ThorsonsAudio.

Gross, R. D. (1999) Psychology: *The Science of Mind and Behaviour*, London: Hodder & Stoughton.

Hadot, P. (1999) *Philosophy as a Way of Life*, Oxford: Blackwell.

Hirst, B. (2002) *Il riso non cresce sugli alberi (Rice does not grow on trees)*, Milano: La Tartaruga.

Jacobs, M. (2002) *Psychodynamic Counselling in Action*, London: Sage.

Kornfield, J. (1994) *Buddha's Little Instruction Book*, New York: Bantam Books.

Laszlo, E. (1978) in Bellino, F. (1988) *Etica della Solidarieta` e Societa` Complessa (Ethics of Solidarity and Complex Society)*, Bari: Levante.

Lazarus, A. A. (1997) *Brief but Comprehensive Psychotherapy*, New York: Springer.

Lawrence, J. in *The Bathroom Inspiration Book*, Saddle River (NJ): Red-Letter Press.

Lefever, R. (2003) *Eating Disorders*, Nonington (Kent): Promis.

Lerner, M. D. and Sheldon, R. D. *Acute Traumatic Stress Management*, New York: AAETS.

Petronio, G. (1977) *Italia Letteraria (History of Italian Literature)*, Roma: Palumbo.

Pinel, J. P. J. (2003) *Biopsychology*, Boston: Allyn and Bacon.

Rossi, V. (2004) *La via del movimento*, Diagaro di Cesena: Macroedizioni

Serra, T. (2005) *Zen Shiatsu,* Milano: Fabbri

Smail, D. (1993) *The Origins of Unhappiness*, London: Harper Collins.

Smail, D. (1998) *How To Survive Without Psychotherapy*, London: Constable.

Thich Nhat Hanh (1997) in Luchinger, T. *Steps of Mindfulness (video)*, Zurich: Luchinger.

Vinay, M.P. (1973) *Hygiene Mentale (Mental Hygiene)*, St Francois Sherbrooke: Editions Paulines.

Articles, papers and training

Burne, J. (2004) *Can this man cure your depression?* The Independent Review, 17 May 2004.

Canter, D. (2002) *The rise and rise of biobabble*, New Scientist, Vol. 173, issue 2336, 30 March 2002, p. 50.

Davidson, R. (2004) in Huppert, Baylis, Keverne (2004) *The science of well-being*, The Psychologist, Vol. 17, No. 1, p. 7.

Deary, I. (2003) *Ten Things I hate about Intelligence Research*, The Psychologist, Vol. 16, No 10, p. 537.

Fairburn, C. G. and Harrison P. J. (2003) *Eating Disorders*, Lancet 2003; 361: 407-16.

Farley, P. (2004) *The anatomy of despair*, New Scientist, Vol. 182, issue 2445, 01 May 2004, p. 42.

Healy (1998) in Palumbo, T. (1999) *A brief Introduction to Essential Psychology*, London (unpublished paper).

Lanza del Vasto (1975), poet, Christian mystic and non-violent activist, Fellowship Magazine, Sept. 1975.

Lawson, W. (2004) *The Glee Club*, Psychology Today, February 2004, p. 34.

Malley-Morrison, K. (2004) *The Evil of Inaction*, Talk given to graduating MA students, Boston University, 16 May 2004.

Morelli, R. & Zerbini E. (2006) *Training in Anti-stress Bodywork,* Rome: Riza Institute.

Palumbo, T. (1999) *A brief Introduction to Essential Psychology*, CMQ, Vol. X, No. 2 (286), London: GCD.

Pointon, C. (2004) *The future of trauma work*, Counselling and Psychotherapy Journal UK, May 2004, p. 10.

Rowe, D. (2001) *The story of depression*, Counselling and Psychotherapy Journal UK, November 2001, p. 5.

Small, M. F. (2002) *The happy fat*, New Scientist, Vol. 175, issue 2357, 24 August 2002, p. 34.

Thernstrom, M. (2001) *Life Without Pain*, The New York Times Magazine, December 16, 2001, New York.

Van der Kolk, B. A. (2002) *EMDR, consciousness and the body*, Boston: The Trauma Center.

Resources

Books

DesMaisons K. (2001) *Potatoes not Prozac*, London: Simon & Schuster.

Kornfield, J. (1994) *Buddha's Little Instruction Book*, New York: Bantam Books.

Tolle, E. (2005) *The Power of Now,* London: Hodder & Stoughton

Professional Organisations

The British Association for Counselling and Psychotherapy (BACP)
BACP House, 35-37 Albert Street, Rugby, CV21 2SG
Tel: 0870 443 5252 - Website: www.bacp.co.uk

The British Psychological Society (BPS)
St Andrews House, 48 Princess Road East, Leicester LE1 7DR
Tel: 0116 254 9568 - Website: www.bps.org.uk

Other National Organisations

The Eating Disorders Association (EDA)
First Floor, Wensum House, 103 Prince of Wales Road, Norwich NR1 1DW
Tel: 0870 770 3256 – Website: www.edauk.com

The National Centre for Eating Disorders (NCFED)
54 New Road, Esher, Surrey, KT10 9NU
Tel: 01372 469 493 – Website: www.eating-disorders.org.uk